Updates on Corticosteroids

Edited by Miroslav Radenkovic

Published in London, United Kingdom

Updates on Corticosteroids
http://dx.doi.org/10.5772/intechopen.105342
Edited by Miroslav Radenkovic

Contributors
Mohammad Ahmadi Dastgerdi, Nafiseh Bavaghar, Aniseh Bavaghar, Virgil I. Stenberg, Ann L. Baldwin, Mohamed Salah S. El-Khooly, Dhoha Ben Salah, Khouloud Boujelbnen, Hanaa Shafiek, Doha Omar Alghamdi, Abdulrahman Alghamdi, Miroslav Radenkovic, Ivana Milicevic

First published in London, United Kingdom, 2023 by IntechOpen
IntechOpen is the global imprint of INTECHOPEN LIMITED, registered in England and Wales, registration number: 11086078, 5 Princes Gate Court, London, SW7 2QJ, United Kingdom

British Library Cataloguing-in-Publication Data
A catalogue record for this book is available from the British Library

Additional hard and PDF copies can be obtained from orders@intechopen.com

Updates on Corticosteroids
Edited by Miroslav Radenkovic
p. cm.
Print ISBN 978-1-83768-625-4
Online ISBN 978-1-83768-626-1
eBook (PDF) ISBN 978-1-83768-627-8

Meet the editor

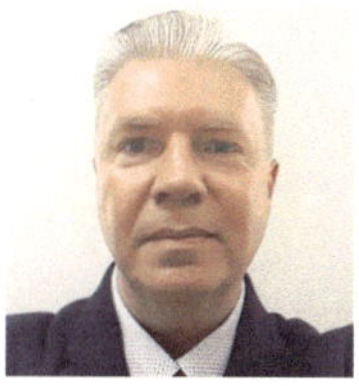

Miroslav Radenković, MD, Ph.D., is a full-time professor who graduated from the Faculty of Medicine, University of Belgrade (FMUB) in 1995. He has been working in the Department of Pharmacology, Clinical Pharmacology and Toxicology, FMUB, since 1996. He received an MS in Pharmacology in 1999, board certification in clinical pharmacology in 2000, a Ph.D. in Medical Sciences in 2004, and a sub-specialization in Clinical Pharmacology - Pharmacotherapy in 2016, all from FMUB. He also obtained an MS in Bioethics from Clarkson University, NYC, USA in 2021. Since 2002, Dr. Radenković has participated in several scientific projects supported by the Ministry of Science – Serbia; the Austrian Science Fund - Vienna, Austria; COST (European Cooperation in Science and Technology); and the NIH Fogarty International Center Project, USA. He is also a member of the Ethics Committee of Serbia.

Contents

Preface

Nearly 70 years after their successful launch into the clinic, corticosteroids are still the most prescribed anti-inflammatory and immunosuppressive pharmacological agents. While corticosteroids are fairly inexpensive and frequently used as a treatment for a variety of pathological conditions, their long-term use is known to be connected with certain adverse effects, including osteoporotic, metabolic, gastrointestinal, or cardiovascular side effects, some of which may even be life-threatening. Corticosteroids are characterized by a complex mechanism of action, with still not fully determined pharmacokinetic and pharmacodynamic differences among various drugs. The benefits and harms of corticosteroids represent an everlasting question in the everyday assessment of the risk-to-benefit ratio during the prescribing process. Nevertheless, new medical indications for corticosteroids are emerging and updating every day.

This book is comprised of two sections on clinical challenges in corticosteroid use and safety and consequences of corticosteroid use. Starting with a comprehensive analysis of corticosteroid use in emergency pathologies, the first section includes valuable contributions on the usage of corticosteroids in musculoskeletal disorders, an assessment of inhaled corticosteroids, and an original study evaluating drug delivery of corticosteroids. The second section evaluates the safe use of cortisol for inflammation disorders, reviews corticosteroid-resistance diseases, and examines low bone mineral density after prolonged corticosteroid replacement therapy.

We hope this volume proves a useful framework for clinicians to further explore and update existing knowledge on corticosteroid use. We also hope that this book will be used as a reference by researchers, medical specialists, teachers, and students. Finally, we express sincere appreciation to all the chapter authors for their enthusiasm and expertise, as well as all the dedicated professionals at IntechOpen for their highly proficient and unconditional support.

Miroslav Radenković, MD, MSc, Ph.D.
Professor,
Faculty of Medicine,
University of Belgrade,
Belgrade, Serbia

Section 1

Clinical Challenges in Corticosteroids Use

Chapter 1

Corticosteroids in Emergency Pathologies

Miroslav Radenković and Ivana Milićević

Abstract

Ever since their discovery in the fifties of the last century, as an anti-inflammatory drugs for the treatment of rheumatoid arthritis, corticosteroids have found a significant place and wide application in various fields of medicine. Their effects are known to be diverse. The most significant ones are the anti-inflammatory, anti-allergic, and immunosuppressive effects. Furthermore, they affect the hematopoietic system. Corticosteroids produce complex metabolic effects by stimulating glyconeogenesis, increasing the uptake of amino acids in the liver and kidneys, and enhancing lipolysis. Given that natural adrenocortical hormones are synthesized under the influence of stress, it is expected that in the emergency situations, where we face vitally endangered patients whose body is under the stress due to respiratory insufficiency or impaired hemodynamics, corticosteroids do have significant place in the treatment. Thus, these drugs are used in the treatment of acute exacerbation of chronic obstructive pulmonary disease and asthma, in anaphylactic reactions, spinal shock, Addisonian crisis, and sepsis. During the COVID-19 pandemic, corticosteroids found their place in certain stages of treatment, as well as in many national protocols for the treatment of COVID-19 patients. Hence, the use of corticosteroids in the emergency pathologies will be reviewed in this chapter.

Keywords: corticosteroids, COPD, asthma, Addisonian crisis, anaphylaxis, sepsis, COVID-19

1. Introduction

From their first discovery, in the fifties of the last century, as anti-inflammatory drugs for the treatment of rheumatoid arthritis, corticosteroids have found a significant place and wide application in various fields of medicine. Natural adrenocortical hormones are steroid molecules that are released from the cortex of the adrenal gland and have numerous physiological functions. These include: (1) glucocorticoids (cortisol), (2) mineralcorticoids (aldosterone), and (3) androgens (dehydroepi-androsterone). Today, numerous synthetic derivatives of natural corticosteroids have been developed, with some enhanced or oppositely reduced pharmacological properties. Glucocorticoids show significant metabolic, anti-inflammatory, immunosuppressive, and vasoconstrictor effects. On the other hand, mineralcorticoids regulate the level of water and salt in the body, help the reabsorption of Na^+ from the kidney tubules, and increase the excretion of K^+. Nevertheless, when we consider the practical application of corticosteroids in various pathological conditions, we usually think of glucocorticoids.

The circadian rhythm of glucocorticoids is influenced by the negative feedback loop of the hypothalamus-pituitary-adrenal cortex. These steroid hormones are synthesized from cholesterol. They achieve their physiological and pharmacological effects through the intracellular glucocorticoid receptor [1]. Initially, they diffuse through the cell membrane and bind to a receptor located on a specific protein. Afterward, this entire complex enters the nucleus and causes the expression of certain genes, responsible for the synthesis of specific proteins. This represents a gene-related and time-consuming mechanism of action. There is also another, faster way of producing the effect, where the glucocorticoid binds to the receptor in the cytoplasm, where protein synthesis is not required, and the effect is achieved after a few minutes of binding to the receptor.

The physiological and pharmacological effects of glucocorticoids are diverse. The most significant ones are related to anti-inflammatory, anti-allergic, and immunosuppressive effects. Consequently, they affect the hematopoietic system, increasing the number of neutrophils while simultaneously decreasing the number of lymphocytes, monocytes, eosinophils, and basophils. They antagonize the effect of vitamin D on the absorption of calcium from the digestive tract. To continue, they stimulate the secretion of hydrochloric acid. These drugs have complex metabolic effects as well, thus stimulating gluconeogenesis, increasing the uptake of amino acids in the liver and kidneys, and enhancing the lipolysis. They also cause catabolic effects in lymphoid and connective tissue and muscles, as well.

Due to the wide range of described effects, a large number of different pathological conditions can be identified where these drugs may be used, including various methods of administration (oral, intravenous, and inhalation). Given that natural adrenocortical hormones are usually synthesized under the influence of stress, in cases where the hypothalamus was stimulated, this endocrine structure releases corticotropin-releasing factor (CRF). Consequently, the pituitary gland releases corticotropin (ACTH) and leads to the release of cortisol, which finally starts a cascade of metabolic processes to overcome the stress. It is expected that in the emergency situations with vitally endangered patients, whose body is under the stress due to the respiratory insufficiency or impaired hemodynamics, the corticosteroids will certainly have an important place in the treatment.

These drugs are used in the treatment of acute exacerbations of chronic obstructive pulmonary disease (COPD) and asthma, in anaphylactic reactions, in spinal shock, and in Addison's disease and related crisis. According to the guidelines for the treatment of sepsis and septic shock from 2017, as well as the revised recommendations from 2021, the corticosteroids are included in the treatment of this serious and urgent condition [2]. During the COVID-19 pandemic, corticosteroids have found their place in certain stages of treatment and were accordingly included in many national protocols for the treatment of COVID-19-positive patients.

In the further segments of this chapter, the most important indications for using glucocorticoids in the emergency pathologies will be addressed.

2. Acute exacerbations of chronic obstructive lung disease

Chronic obstructive pulmonary disease (COPD) is characterized by limited (reduced) airflow in the airways. The obstruction is progressive and related to the inflammatory process caused by harmful particles and gases from the external environment. Smokers and mostly people over 40 years of age were linked to the COPD.

It is the third most common cause of death in the world and the seventh cause of reduced overall health ability [3]. According to data from the World Health Organization (WHO) from 2011, only in the USA, there were about 13 million adults being treated from the COPD [4]. The main symptoms of COPD include choking, coughing, and expectoration of the purulent contents. Acute exacerbation of the disease obligatory implies the need for the additional therapy and in some cases hospitalization, and it clearly affects the progression of the disease and mortality. Exacerbations of COPD are most often associated with infection, inhalation of air pollution, and the influence of other chronic diseases that the patient is suffering from. Given the heterogeneity of the disease exacerbation causes, the basic form of COPD treatment is related to the causal therapy against the causative agent, modulation of the overall body's response, and the maintenance of the patient's respiratory and hemodynamic status.

Corticosteroids are present in all protocols for the treatment of acute COPD, but determining the most effective dose and duration of therapy is still a subject of research. They are used as intravenous, oral, and inhalation therapy. They improve ventilation and gas exchange, as shown by pulmonary function tests; also reduce dyspnea; and, finally, speed up the recovery and duration of hospital treatment.

Systemic corticosteroids have been the standard therapy in COPD exacerbations for many years. Of course, long-term use of glucocorticoids is an independent risk factor for increased mortality in patients with COPD. This is mainly due to a number of possible side effects and the impact of therapy on associated diseases. The *Reduce* study showed that the therapy with 40 mg of prednisone intravenously for 5 days was as effective as 14-day therapy in terms of repeated exacerbations [5]. The latest guidelines of the European Respiratory and American Chest Association favor a shorter treatment period (less than 14 days) and emphasize the use of oral preparations over the systemic ones. Even for patients who are hospitalized for the treatment of exacerbations, a short-term oral therapy is recommended [6]. Several studies have shown better efficacy of short-term therapy, as well as favorable pharmacokinetics of this type of treatment, which enables adequate drug bioavailability. In addition to systemic and oral therapy, inhalation therapy with corticosteroids, in combination with long-acting bronchodilators, was shown to be effective, too [7].

Today, clinicians are turning to the latest guidelines from the *GOLD* study, which represents the Global Strategy for the Diagnosis, Treatment, and Prevention of COPD, revised in 2019 [8]. The *GOLD* study emphasizes an individual approach, based on the severity of symptoms, risk of exacerbation, comorbidities, adverse effects, response to therapy, and availability of medication. This is precisely why the number of eosinophils is determined for each patient, because the anti-inflammatory effect of corticosteroids depends on how much inflammation plays a role in the pathogenesis of the disease. Recent studies have shown that the number of eosinophils is a direct predictor of the effectiveness of corticosteroids in preventing future exacerbations. Therefore, an individual pharmacological treatment plan must be applied for each patient, both for the disease and for an emergency, such as an exacerbation, still based on comorbidities, severity of symptoms, risk of side effects, hemodynamic, and respiratory status.

3. Acute asthma exacerbations

Asthma is a chronic inflammation of the airways that causes their hypersensitivity to various factors from the external environment. In fact, they provoke a narrowing of the airways, which in turn causes discomfort in the form of a feeling of shortness of breath, coughing, and wheezing in the chest. The disease can occur in young children, and it can also develop in the elderly. There are numerous causes, recognized as external and internal ones. The external ones include air pollution, allergens in the air, pollen, industrialization, internal genetic predisposition, a diet with use of additives, maternal smoking during pregnancy, and so on. All these factors lead to airway inflammation, further increased mucus production, airway wall remodeling, and bronchial hypersensitivity. Given that inflammation has a key role in the pathogenesis of the disease, the main goal in the treatment of asthma is to control the symptoms and signs of inflammation in order to avoid future exacerbations.

An acute asthma attack is an episode of progressive suffocation, shortness of breath, coughing, and wheezing in the chest. According to some authors, an acute asthma attack is one specific condition that requires the use of systemic corticosteroids [9].

It has been established that corticosteroids reduce inflammation in the airways. They are most commonly used in the form of inhalation preparations in the chronic therapy of asthma as well as systemically when needed in severe exacerbation episodes. The recommendation in all guidelines for the treatment of acute asthma attack is to repeat the inhaled dose of a drug and if there is no improvement, to introduce systemic therapy. As with COPD, the preference is given to oral preparations, 50 mg of prednisolone for 5–7 days [10]. As previously confirmed, a short-term treatment is considered to be more effective [11]. It is recommended to introduce the oral preparation in the first hour of the attack. Oral preparations are recommended in exacerbations, as well as maintenance therapy in patients with a severe form of the disease, which accounts for about 10% of patients. Of course, the use of oral and systemic corticosteroids can be associated with a number of side effects. This is why the recommendations direct us to use systemic corticosteroids only for 5–7 days during acute exacerbation. In a large cohort study, Vorham et al. [12] showed that the use of oral corticosteroids in Great Britain is far higher than recommended, in terms of doses (more than 7.5 mg/dL) and duration of administration, wherein the excessive administration was explained by the low price of these drugs.

A special form of exacerbation of the disease is the status asthmaticus, a vitally threatening condition with hypoxia, hypercapnia, and a high risk of developing acute respiratory insufficiency. The recommendation for the treatment of this condition is, in addition to oxygen support, bronchodilators and 125 mg methylprednisolone intravenously [13].

Finally, it has to be underlined that in addition to unwanted effects of corticosteroids, there is also a problem of effectiveness in some patients, in the sense that not all patients have a good therapeutic response, which means that an individual approach is needed. Therefore, the balance between the efficacy and safety of therapy must be established for each and every patient.

4. Anaphylaxis

Anaphylaxis is a severe allergic reaction, which has a rapid onset and development of symptoms and can cause an anaphylactic shock with a possible fatal outcome. Allergic reactions can be induced by medicines, food ingredients, insect bites, and so on. Visual changes rapidly occur at the point of an allergen entry, followed by itching, urticaria of the skin, angioedema, bronchospasm, rhinorrhea, gastrointestinal disorders, a drop in arterial tension, and, if not responded to in time, an overall shock. The first step in treatment would be to administer epinephrine.

Glucocorticoids are often given in anaphylaxis, but there is a little evidence of their effectiveness. Due to the specific mechanism of action, which includes intracellular position of the respective receptors, their effect may take several hours to be fully developed. So, these drugs would not be able to act on the initial signs and symptoms of anaphylaxis. However, one of the reasons for their widespread use in this disorder is to prevent the second (so-called protracted) phase of an anaphylactic reaction, which sometimes may exist or occur even after several hours. Nonetheless, in the recent literature, there are several studies that did not confirm the previous notion. Hence, the use of glucocorticoids can be possibly justified in patients who are hospitalized for anaphylaxis, in order to further prevent bronchospasm, or who are already being treated from COPD and asthma.

In 2021, the Resuscitation Council of Great Britain published the new guidelines for the care and treatment of anaphylaxis that support the complete exclusion of the use of glucocorticoids. There was reportedly little evidence to support that glucocorticoids prevent the delayed response. In some studies, it has even been shown that the use of these drugs was associated with greater mobility, or increased hospitalization, in the case of prehospital administration. The explanations suggested that perhaps the administration of glucocorticoids actually delayed the administration of epinephrine, which should be the first drug of choice in this case [14, 15].

5. Spinal shock

Spinal shock, occurring after spinal cord injury, is a special pathological condition characterized by the loss of all neurological activity below the level of injury. These would include the loss of motor, sensory, reflex, and autonomic functions. It starts 30–60 minutes after the spinal cord injury and can last up to 6 weeks after the injury. It can lead to permanent disability.

Until recently, methylprednisolone was widely used in the early stages of treatment after the spinal cord injury, namely, in the first 8 hours. In recent years, more and more studies have shown that there is no difference between patients that received methylprednisolone and the placebo group, especially in terms of the motor response. The side effects are unfortunately numerous [16]. In animal models, the follow-up studies provided specific evidence at the molecular level, as well. Thus, Nelson et al. [17] showed in their research using a fish model that glucocorticoids inhibited neuron regeneration by directly acting on ependymal glial cells, independently of microglia.

Considering the severity of the clinical presentation that exists in a spinal cord injury, as well as a series of side effects related to corticosteroids, more studies are needed to examine the exact relationship between the risks and benefits of using these drugs in this specific condition.

6. Addisonian crisis

Addison's disease is a rare chronic condition that occurs when the adrenal glands are unable to provide sufficient amounts of hormones (glucocorticoids, mineralocorticoids, and androgens). Consequently, therapeutic hormone replacement is necessary. Addison's disease is also called primary adrenal insufficiency. Given that quoted hormones participate in the metabolism of water and electrolytes, and are also important for producing energy, this is a clinically difficult condition that can initially occur its most serious form—adrenal crisis. The patient is vitally endangered with a severe clinical picture of arterial hypotension, dehydration, abdominal pain, nausea, and vomiting. Addisonian crisisis not such a common condition, but it is linked with a high mortality rate, as much as 45% [18]. The most common causes of adrenal gland insufficiency are autoimmune disease, then tumor infiltrations, and infarctions or hemorrhages within the glands, and so on. When the disease develops gradually, it is very difficult to establish the correct diagnosis, because the symptoms and signs are general and nonspecific, including malaise, weakness, muscle pain, loss of body mass, or hyperpigmentation on the skin.

Primary adrenal insufficiency occurs as a result of disturbed function of the adrenal gland itself, primarily in an autoimmune disease, severe infection, or cessation of the cortisol production in newborns due to congenital adrenal hyperplasia. Secondary adrenal insufficiency occurs due to dysfunction of the hypothalamus-pituitary-adrenal axis. Inadequate stimulation of the adrenal cortex occurs due to lack of adrenocorticotropic Hormone (ACTH). This condition frequently occurs associated with tumors of the pituitary gland, surgical interventions in that anatomical region, as well as after its radiation [19]. It is very important for clinicians to clarify whether a primary or a secondary adrenal insufficiency is present, because in the primary adrenal insufficiency, all the hormones produced by the adrenal cortex are absent while in the secondary insufficiency, only the hormones secreted under control of ACTH (cortisol and sex hormones). Substitution of aldosterone, which is controlled by the renin-angitensin system, is not required.

Addisonian crisis can also occur in people with adrenal insufficiency being on substitution therapy with glucocorticoids but experiencing specific circumstances, such as trauma, infection, increased effort, pregnancy, surgical interventions, and so on. It has to be underlined that the Addisonian crisis is an urgent endocrinological condition, where the prompt diagnosis and initiation of therapy is of crucial importance, since if the adequate therapy would not be started on time, a fatal outcome can occur.

Initial treatment in Addisonian crisis involves intravascular volume replacement with the crystalloid isotonic solutions and the correction of hypoglycemia by using 5% glucose solution. A correction of hormonal status by using glucocorticoids and mineralcorticoids is required, as well. Thus, in an adrenal crisis, it is necessary to immediately prescribe 100 mg intravenous hydrocortisone and then to continue with 50–100 mg intravenously every 6 hours during 1 day. In children, the recommended dose is 50 mg/m^2, with maximum of 100 mg. Given that quoted doses of glucocorticoids have minimal mineralocorticoid effects, it is not necessary additionally to prescribe fludrocortisone (a mineralcorticoid) at this time.

There are still challenges existing in treating Addisonian crisis. First of all, there are no adequate biomarkers that would show us the exact levels of cortisol in the tissues. It is encouraging that there are some studies that may provide us with a certain precision in determination of cortisol in hair, saliva, and subcutaneous fat tissue [20]. It is very difficult to prescribe quite precise individual effective dose, because the levels of glucocorticoids in the blood are under different influences, and of course, there is also an existing receptor polymorphism, which needs to be considered. It is also challenging to establish how much it is necessary to increase the initial doses of glucocorticoids during the treatment that are given as a substitution in a different setting of stress reactions. Although there are studies that could investigate this problem in clear situations of infections, surgical interventions, and trauma, it is quite another thing to determine how much glucocorticoids we need during an emotional stress. Therefore, more studies are needed to help us in determining a precise individual therapeutic regimen for Addisonian crisis.

7. Sepsis

Sepsis is a life-threatening condition accompanied with organic dysfunction, which is caused by an inadequate response of the body to an infection. Considering the high incidence and mortality, as well as long-term treatment in intensive care units associated with high costs, the sepsis has become a global problem in the recent decades. For these reasons, the scientific community has been working for a long time to develop common guidelines for the prevention, rapid detection, and treatment of sepsis through the Surviving Sepsis Campaign guide. The last recommendations were revised in 2021. The guidelines help in faster recognition of sepsis, earlier initiation of antibiotic therapy, and maintenance of the patient's hemodynamic status, respiratory support, and additional therapy.

Patients with sepsis have an increased heart and respiratory rate, decreased systolic pressure, disturbed consciousness, and elevated body temperature. Septic shock can occur very quickly, represented by circulatory, cellular, and metabolic instability, and it arise with a mean arterial pressure (MAP) of less than 65 mmHg and a lactate level of more than 2 mmol/L [21]. For that reason, it is of crucial importance regarding the sepsis therapy to establish hemodynamic stability and a tissue perfusion as soon as possible. There are clear guidelines for the amount and type of infusion solutions, as well as for prescribing vasopressors. The recommendations for the treatment of sepsis from 2016 advised the use of hydrocortisone intravenously only in patients who cannot reach hemodynamic stability despite fluid replacement therapy and the inclusion of the recommended vasopressor drugs.

The latest recommendations from 2021 state that intravenous hydrocortisone should be included for all patients being in septic shock and required vasopressor support. Hence, hydrocortisone is to be prescribed in a dose of 200 mg intravenously daily, 50 mg every 6 hours, or in a continuous infusion. Since the previous guidelines were instituted, three large studies have been published on the use of corticosteroids in the treatment of sepsis [22, 23]. Rigard et al. [24] also showed in their meta-analysis that systemic corticosteroids accelerated recovery from shock and shortened the time of vasopressor use. However, in this analysis, it was established that corticosteroids increase neuromuscular weakness, and there is still no clear connection between their use and the impact on mortality, too. So, taking all together previous facts into account, in an attempt to balance the pros and cons, these drugs are still to be included in the recommendations for the treatment of sepsis.

Given that the pathogenesis of sepsis is based on an inadequate immune response, it is logical that clinicians have long been trying to include corticosteroids as drugs with anti-inflammatory effects in the regular therapy. Liang et al. [25] showed in their meta-analysis that corticosteroids had no effect on mortality after 28 days or on long-term mortality, but they did detect some reduction in in-hospital mortality. They also showed that corticosteroids prolong time the patient is without vasopressor and ventilatory support as well as increase the incidence of side effects, such as hyperglycemia and hypernatremia. Moreover, the use of corticosteroids was associated with a shorter duration of hospitalization in the covered randomized studies. Nevertheless, the proper timing of systemic corticosteroids use in sepsis is still under investigation. This all lead us to the conclusion that more studies are needed to help clarifying the individual steps in the pathophysiological process of sepsis so that clinicians could decide on the type of therapy and the precise timing for each individual drug.

8. COVID-19

At the end of 2019, a number of patients with pneumonia of unknown etiology appeared in the Chinese city of Wuhan. It was quickly established that the causative agent of coronavirus disease (COVID-19) is a virus from the Coronaviridae family, which was named Novel Coronavirus, that is, SARS-Cov-2 (Severe Acute Respiratory Coronavirus). The disease has been proved to be extremely contagious; it quickly took the form of an epidemic, so afterward, on March 11, 2020, the World Health Organization (WHO) announced the beginning of a pandemic. Quick diagnosis was difficult due to the non-specificity of symptoms and laboratory findings. The therapy included antiviral drugs, anticoagulants, corticosteroids, biological and multivitamin therapy, as well as oxygen support.

At the beginning of the pandemic, the use of corticosteroids in the treatment of COVID-19 had a controversial character. Given that it was discovered early that the disease leads to impairment in regulation of the immune response and excessive production of cytokines, it was logical that drugs with an anti-inflammatory and immunosuppressive effects would have a therapeutic effect. It has been later shown that corticosteroids were useful in patients who were on oxygen support, especially those on mechanical ventilation, and these drugs should be avoided in those with a milder form of the disease or with specific comorbidities, due to a series of possible drug-induced unwanted effects [26].

Many randomized studies have shown that corticosteroids reduced mortality in COVID-19 [27]. This led the WHO to include corticosteroids in the guidelines for the treatment of patients with a severe form of the disease [28]. Accordingly, corticosteroids have also been shown to reduce mortality and the duration of mechanical ventilation in affected patients [29].

The large randomized study RECOVERY [30] investigated the effectiveness of dexamethasone administration in patients with COVID-19. The results showed that mortality in those who received dexamethasone was significantly lower compared to the group that received the other proposed therapy, especially in patients who were on mechanical ventilation or had an oxygen support. The mortality in those who did not require oxygen support did not differ from patients who were without corticosteroids. Also, the study showed that in those who did not take corticosteroids and were on oxygen support, deterioration in terms of the need for mechanical ventilation occurred more often.

The WHO provided a prospective meta-analysis of existing research on the treatment of COVID-19, the so-called REACT study [31]. The analysis showed that mortality was lower in the groups of patients who received corticosteroids. Mortality did not differ between the dexamethasone and the hydrocortisone groups. There was no difference to in terms of the amount of dose, as well. This meta-analysis showed that the success of therapy depended on the severity of the clinical presentation. Namely, the efficacy of the corticosteroids use was more pronounced in the group that presented severe clinical features with the need for oxygen support or mechanical ventilation. This meta-analysis also showed the effect of corticosteroids on prolonging the elimination of the virus through the mucous membranes of the nasopharynx and oropharynx. This resulted in prolonging the time of the positive result of the PCR test and was explained by the suppression of the immune response. Based on the previous facts, the WHO made adjusted recommendations for the treatment of COVID-19 infection and included corticosteroids in standard therapy. The European Respiratory Society gave a strong recommendation for the systemic use of corticosteroids, as well [32].

Acknowledgements

This research was funded by the Ministry of Science and Technological Development of the Republic of Serbia; Grant No. 200110.

Author details

Miroslav Radenković[1]* and Ivana Milićević[2]

1 Department of Pharmacology, Clinical Pharmacology and Toxicology, Faculty of Medicine, University of Belgrade, Belgrade, Serbia

2 Department of Emergency Medicine, Emergency Center Belgrade, University Clinical Center of Serbia, Belgrade, Serbia

*Address all correspondence to: miroslav.radenkovic@med.bg.ac.rs

References

[1] Ramamoorthy S, Cidlowski JA. Corticosteroids–Mechanisms of action in health and disease. Rheumatic Diseases Clinics of North America. 2016;**42**(1):15-31

[2] Mirijello A, Tosoni A. On behalf of the internal medicine sepsis study group. New strategies for treatment of sepsis. Medicina (Kaunas, Lithuania). 2020;**56**(10):E527

[3] Heron M. Deaths: Leading causes for 2017. National Vital Statistics Reports. 2019;**68**(6):1-77

[4] World Health Organization. The top 10 causes of death. 2018

[5] Leuppi JD, Shuetz P, Bingisser R, et al. Short-term vs conventional glucocorticoid therapy in acute exacerbations of chronic obstructive pulmonary disease. Journal of the American Medical Association. 2013;**309**(21):2223-2231

[6] Wedzicha JA, Miravittles M, Hurst JR, et al. Management of COPD exacerbations: European Respiratory Society guidline. The European Respiratory Journal. 2017;**49**:1600791

[7] Nakamura Y, Tamaoki J, Nagase H, Yamaguchi M, et al. Japanese Society of Allergology. Japanese guidelines for adult asthma. 2020. Allergology International. 2020;**69**(4):519-548

[8] Singh D, Agusti A, Anzueto A, Barnes PJ, Bourbeau J, Celli BR, et al. Global strategy for the diagnosis, management, and prevention of chronic obstructive lung disease: The GOLD science committee report 2019. European Respiratory Journal. 2019;**53**(5):1900164. DOI: 10.1183/13993003.00164-2019

[9] Fuhlbrigge A, Peden D, Apter AJ, Boushey HA, Camargo CA Jr, Germ J, et al. Asthma outcomes: Exacerbations. The Journal of Allergy and Clinical Immunology. 2012;**129**:s34-s48

[10] Global Initiative for Asthma Management and Prevention (GINA) Difficult –to-Treat and Severe Asthma in Adolescent and Adult Patients, Diagnosis and Management. 2019. Available from: www.ginasthma.org

[11] Price D, Castro M, et al. Short-course systematic corticosteroids in asthma: Striking balance between efficancy and safety. European Respiratory Review. 2020;**29**(155):190151

[12] Vorham J, Menzies Gow A, Tran TN, et al. Longitudinal systemic corticosteroid utilisation for asthma and other disease in the United Kngdom from 1990 to 2018: A population based cohort analysis. Thorax. 2021;**76**(supl. 1):A21

[13] Chakraborty RK, Basnet S. Status Asthmaticus. 2022 Oct 10. In: StatPearls. Treasure Island (FL): StatPearls Publishing; 2022

[14] Nagata S, Ohbe H, Matsui H, Fushimi K, Yasunaga H. Glucocorticoids and rates of biphasic reactions in patients with adrenaline treated anaphylaxis: A propensity score matching analysis. International Archives of Allergy and Immunology. 2022;**183**(9):939-945

[15] Whyte AF, Soar J, Dodd A, Hughes A, Sargant N, Turner PJ. Emergency treatment of anaphylaxis; concise clinical guidance. Clinical Medicine (London, England). 2022;**22**(4):332-339

[16] Liu Z, Yang Y, He L, Pang M, Luo C, Liu B, et al. High-dose

methylprednisolone for acute traumatic spinal cord injury: A meta-analysis. Neurology. 2019;**93**(9):e841-e850

[17] Nelson CM, Lennon VA, Lee H, Krug RG 2nd, Kamalova A, Madigan NN, et al. Glucocorticoids target ependymal glia and inhibit repair of the injured spinal cord. Frontiers in Cell and Developmental Biology. 2019;**7**:56

[18] Betterle C, Pressoto F, Furmaniak J. Epidemiology, pathogenesis and diagnosis of Addison s disease in adults. Journal of Endocrinological Investigation. 2019;**42**(12):1407-1433

[19] Dineen R, Thompson CJ, Sherlock M. Adrenal crisis: Prevention and management in adult patients. Therapeutic Advances in Endocrinology and Metabolism. 2019;**10**:2042018819848218

[20] Claessen KM, Andela CD, Biermasz NR, Pereira AM. Clinical unmet needs in the treatment of adrenal crisis: Importance of the patient's perspective. Frontiers in Endocrinology. 2021;**12**:701365

[21] Huang M, Cai S, Su J. The pathogenesis of sepsis and potential therapeutic targets. International Journal of Molecular Sciences. 2019;**20**(21):5376

[22] Annane D, Renault A, Brun-Buisson C, et al. CRICS-TRIGGERSEP network. Hydrocortisone plus fludrocortisone for adults with septic shock. The New England Journal of Medicine. 2018;**378**:809-818

[23] Venkatesh B, Finfer S, Cohen J, et al. Adjunctive glucocorticoid therapy in patients with septic shock. The New England Journal of Medicine. 2018;**378**:797-808

[24] Rygard SL, Butler E, Granholm A, et al. Low-dose corticosteroids for adult patients with septic shock: A systematic review with meta-analysis and trial sequential analysis. Intensive Care Medicine. 2018;**44**:1003-1016

[25] Liang H, Song H, Zhai R, Song G, Li H, Ding X, et al. Corticosteroids for treating sepsis in adult patients: A systematic review and meta-analysis. Frontiers in Immunology. 2021;**12**:709155

[26] Milenkovic M, Dukic M, Brajkovic M, Klasnja S, Toskovic B, Zdravkovic M. Primenakortikosteroida u terapiji COVID -19 infekcije. Serbian Journal of Anesthesia and Intensive Therapy. 2021;**43**(5-6):85-96

[27] WHO Rapid Evidence Appraisal for COVID-19 Therapies (REACT) Working Group, JAC S, Murthy S, et al. Association between administration of systemic corticosteroids and mortality among critically ill patients with COVID-19: A meta-analysis. The Journal of the American Medical Association. 2020

[28] Lamontagne F, Agarwal A, Rochwerg B, Siemieniuk RA, Agoritsas T, Askie L, et al. A living WHO guideline on drugs for COVID-19. BMJ. 2020;**370**:m3379

[29] Chadhuri D, Sasaki K, Karkar A, Sharif S, Lewis K, Mammen MJ, et al. Corticosteroids in COVID-19 and non-COVID 19 ARDS: A systematic review and meta-analysis. Intensive Care Medicine. 2021;**47**(5):521-537

[30] Horby P, Lim WS, Emberson JR, Mafham M, Bell JL, Linsell L, et al. On behalf of the RECOVERY collaborative group. Dexamethasone in hospitalized patients with COVID-19. The New England Journal of Medicine. 2021;**384**(8):693-704

[31] The WHO Rapid Evidence Appraisal for COVID-19 Therapies (REACT) working Group. Association

between administration of systemic corticosteroids and mortality among critically Ill patients With COVID-19: A meta-analysis. The Journal of the American Medical Association. 2020;**324**(13):1330-1341

[32] Agoristas T, John Adabie Appiah J, Arabi Y, Blumberg L, Calfee C, Cao B, et al. Corticosteroids for COVID-19-Living guidance (World Health Organization). 2020. Available from: https://apps.who.int/iris/handle/

Chapter 2

Usage of Corticosteroids in Musculoskletal Disorders

Mohammad Ahmadi-Dastgerdi, Nafiseh Bavaghar and Aniseh Bavaghar

Abstract

Corticosteroids are one of the most important anti-inflammatory substances that are used for many conditions. Although oral form of corticosteroids has many side effects, they are used to cure systemic diseases. Local injection of corticosteroids can be beneficial in many conditions such as mononeuropathies, degenerative joint diseases (DJD), tenosynovitis, and canal stenosis with fewer side effects and better efficacy in site of pathology.

Keywords: corticosteroid, ultrasonography, mononeuropathy, tendinitis, osteoarthritis

1. Introduction

We normally know corticosteroids as steroids that are one of the most important anti-inflammatory medications that are used to manage a broad variety of diseases.

This substance normally secrets by adrenal glands in response to different modules of stress and plays a very important role in humans daily life.

Different forms of this medicine such as prednisone, methylprednisolone, triamcinolone, hydrocortisone, and cortisone are used to manage a broad variety of musculoskeletal diseases. For example, the oral form of corticosteroids is used to cure systemic diseases like rheumatoid arthritis (RA) [1]. In chronic use of oral corticosteroids, the side effects are common and serious from time to time, like high blood pressure, edema as a reason of fluid retention, mood changes, weight gain, and facial features changes (moon face), ophthalmic problems like glaucoma and cataract, and high blood sugar that can exacerbate the existing diabetes and also cause overt diabetes and insulin-resistant patients, increased incidence of opportunistic fungal infections like *Candida albicans* and mucormycosis and serious infections like tuberculosis and also common bacterial, viral, and fungal infections and sometimes causes some skin conditions like frequent bruising and delayed wound healing [2].

Most of the patients who suffer from joint degenerative diseases like osteoarthritis (OA) and complain from severe pain and decreased quality of life are middle-aged and old people, and the side effects of corticosteroids intake are severally dangerous for them.

One of the very important side effects of prolonged oral corticosteroid intake is osteoporosis that limits the use of the medicine for old people. On account of this, patients already experience some diminished bone tissue mineralization due to various reasons like malnutrition and systemic diseases. In these patients that include a large number of musculoskeletal patients to allocate pain and inflammatory joint conditions, the local injection of corticosteroids can be beneficial [1, 2].

In this treatment, there are no such side effects as the systemic use, and on the other hand the medicine can act on the problematic area, like injecting the injectable form of triamcinolone in the joint space. Usually to eliminate patient's pain in this treatment, corticosteroid is mixed with local anesthetic agents like lidocaine and is injected directly in the joint space either landmark-guided or sonographic-guided [3–12].

Although this injection is way easier in large- and medium-sized joints for the operator to perform, it can also be used in smaller joints like metacarpophalangeal (MCP) and shows significant improvements in discomfort and swelling.

In this chapter, the types of intra-articular injections and their clinical application are discussed.

2. Corticosteroids application in musculoskeletal diseases

2.1 Corticosteroids application in carpal tunnel syndrome

The carpal tunnel syndrome (CTS) is referred to a condition in which the median nerve (that enters from forearm to the wrist) is stuck in the carpal tunnel. This nerve is responsible for innervation parts of thenar muscles and provide sensation for 3½ of the lateral fingers of the hand. After the nerve trap and pressure upon it, patient experiences symptoms like numbness in 3½ of the lateral fingers and in severe cases feeling of weakness and sometimes hand muscles atrophy; for example, the thenar prominence atrophy is initiated.

This condition is found in 5% of the population mostly in middle-aged women (F to M ratio: 3 to 1) and is related to age, weight, hypothyroidism, diabetes, repetitive wrist flexion, and pregnancy. This condition is divided to three different forms based on clinical presentation, electromyography, and nerve conduction velocity (EMG-NCV) and sonographic findings to mid, moderate, or severe [3, 4].

In mild and moderate form, the application of injectable corticosteroid can be used to decrease pain and adhesion on the nerve and tendon sheath around the nerve. This results in pressure sensation on the nerve and mends the patient's signs and symptoms. In severe form, the noninvasive treatment is used first and if it was not successful or thenar atrophy (the medial prominence of the palm) is present, the invasive treatment is recommended which is surgery to cut the transverse ligament on the nerve and suture it on a higher distance [3, 4].

2.2 Joint arthritis

Osteoarthritis is a degenerative joint problem that occurs with aging, wrong lifestyle, persistent and unsuitable use of joints, obesity, sports, and traumatic injury.

In this condition, the joint cartilage which has no nerve innervation and plays a very important role in easing movement and prohibiting the head of the bones from erosion is damaged and absorbed. After the initiation of arthritis process, patient experiences a progressive pain which gets worse by time and highly affects patient's quality of life [13]. Recently, joint replacement which is aggressive but very effective method to manage arthritis is widely used for big joints like hip and knee. In this method, the joint and the heads of bones are cut and replaced with an artificial metal joint that can eliminate the pain and stiffness and other symptoms of arthritis.

This surgery like other surgical methods requires post-op care and use of other medications to avoid infection and clot accumulation due to motionlessness [14].

After the operation, strengthening of involved muscles in joint movement by routine workouts is highly recommended.

In mild and moderate and some major forms that patients cannot undergo surgery (like patients with decompensated heart failure, pulmonary edema, and other underlying conditions), arthritis in a joint that there is no proper way to replace it yet or when patient does not accept surgery, intra-articular injections can be beneficial. Various medicines can serve this purpose like hyaluronic acid gel (to improve joint surfaces to slide on each other and reduce erosion on bone ends), Botox, and platelet-rich plasma (PRP).

One of the very common medications which can work alone or mixed with hyaluronic acid is corticosteroid.

Corticosteroid is very helpful in mending arthritis symptoms, and patient is pain-free for about 2–3 months.

Compared to corticosteroids, hyaluronic acid takes longer to effect but reduces the pain for about 6 months, while PRP does it for 12 months [13]. In this time, patient can strength the muscles around the joint and have normal daily activities pain-free. Side effects of this kind of injections are septic arthritis (due to bacterial infiltration from skin while performing the injection) and bleeding (in coagulopathic patients) which can be prevented with a good medical history taking before starting the procedure and proper disinfection of the injection area.

In severe and progressive cases, the injection needs to repeat every 3–6 months, and because the side effects are few and preventable, intra-articular injections with corticosteroid seem to be harmless and beneficial. This injection with corticosteroid is permitted three times a year [5].

2.3 Tenosynovitis

Tenosynovitis is referred to a group of condition that causes tendonitis and synovitis. De Quervain is one of this conditions that causes inflammation on tendons of extensor tendon of fingers (abductor pollicis longus and extensor pollicis brevis). Patients experience pain while grabbing on objects, fisting, and rotating the hand. To mend this inflammatory condition, first-line treatment is local corticosteroid injection in problematic tendon sheath. In different studies, it was proved that this injection clearly makes the symptoms better compared to placebo in short term [6].

2.4 Adhesive capsulitis

In this condition, severe stiffness in shoulder joint with pain and reduced range of motion (ROM) is present. There are three phases to this condition: first, the pain is dominant and local intra-articular corticosteroid injection can be beneficial. Then in the second phase, the pain decreases and ROM is reduced. In this step, greater volume of local intra-articular volume injection (attenuated corticosteroid with normal salin) can be useful. In third phase, there is a significant improvement in ROM. This condition is referred to as self-limited, and with physiotherapy and over the counter (OTC) analgesics the symptoms are improved to some extent.

Sometimes, patients complain from severe continuous pain; in this case, the intra-articular and sub-acromial corticosteroid injections are useful. If symptoms do not improve over the use of injectable corticosteroid, surgical methods are indicated to cut the fibrous bundles [7, 8].

2.5 Medial and lateral epicondylitis

In lateral epicondylitis (tennis elbow), the origin of wrist extensor muscles in elbow area is inflamed due to continuous use. Most of the patients recover after time pass and physiotherapy, nonsteroidal anti-inflammatory drugs (NSAIDs), other anti-inflammatory medication, and resting the muscles of the area.

In case of severe pain and limited daily activities, local injections, especially steroids, are a potent and valid anti-inflammatory agent that can help, although relapse happens in 50% of the cases after injection [9].

Medial epicondylitis (Golf elbow) is persistent pain in medial epicondyle. In this condition, like the lateral epicodylitis, the use of corticosteroid injection can help, but relapsing is common and the use of dextrose prolotherapy and PRP can benefit the patient for a longer period [10].

2.6 Trigger finger

In this condition, finger Pulley A1 that reasons smooth tendon movements in flexor digitorum superficialis and profound muscles is inflamed and holds the finger back while moving. Treatment can either involve surgery to cut pulley or local corticosteroid injection. Corticosteroid injection shows a significant improvement in patient's symptoms, so it is recommended in most of the patients suffering this condition [11].

2.7 Greater trochanter bursitis

One of the very important differential diagnoses in lateral hip discomforts is inflammation of the burse on the greater trochanter. To cure it NSAIDs, physiotherapy and corticosteroid injection is recommended, the later can benefit the patient faster and better [12].

2.8 Facet joints injection

Facet joints are on both sides of each vertebrae and connect each thoracic, cervical, and lumbar vertebrae to its upper and lower. Arthritis or inflammation in this joint causes pain in spine. Corticosteroid accompanied by anesthetic agents' injection in this joint is an easy procedure which is usually done by sonography or fluoroscopy guidance. The injection itself means no harm, and patient experiences the least convalescence period [15, 16].

Corticosteroid onset of effect in this type of injection is commonly 3–7 days and remains for couple of months. This treatment becomes so popular lately, since it is both noninvasive and effective in reducing pain and symptoms. This injection is advantageous on the other hand. If patient feels a significant improvement, the other techniques that have constant effects are recommended such as facet neurolysis injection and rhizolysis [15, 16].

2.9 Epidural injection to treat disk herniation and canal constriction

In cases like herniated disk, slipped vertebrae, listhesis, joint synovial cyst, spinal ligaments thickening due to spinal arthritis, epidural corticosteroid injection is useful.

In this method, the medication is injected by interlaminar on the fatty layer on the spine or transforaminal or caudal (with a greater volume). This method is very popular between clinicians and patients and provides a good improvement in patents' pain. Side effects include steroid flush as profuse heat sensation for couple of days, sleep disorders, anxiety, edema, and rarely an increase in pain for the few first days. From time to time, patient experiences a provisional paralysis in lower organs after the injection which goes away after the lidocaine or other anesthetic agents effects wear off. To increase the effect of injection, rehabilitation after performing the injection is very important [17]. Two days after the injection, patient needs complete rest, and 2 weeks later relative rest is recommended. After corticosteroid injection to prevent the joints pain, cryotherapy is indicated.

3. Conclusions

Corticosteroids are used in a wide range of disorders, and local injection is curative in mononeuropathies and inflammatory conditions such as de Quervain tenosynovitis and has temporary pain relief in DJDs and spinal canal stenosis.

Conflict of interest

The authors declare no conflict of interest.

Appendices and nomenclature

Adrenal gland	two glands which are located above kidneys and secrete lots of essential hormones including Aldosterone, corticosteroid, sex hormones, and epinephrine
Glaucoma	an eye disease that can cause serious visual impairment like blindness and decreased vision acuity
Cataract	when the lens of the eye becomes cloudy
Candida albicans	a form of fungal infection that can cause mild skin infection to severe life-threatening systemic infection in case of immunocompromised patients
Mucormycosis	an invasive fungal infection than produce serious life-threatening infection in form of severe respiratory infection and black scars around the mouth and nose (skin involvement)
EMG-NCV	a noninvasive diagnostic procedure that the physician can check the electrical activity of muscles and nerves

Platelet-rich plasma (PRP)	a concentration of patient's own platelet that is excluded from complete blood
Synovium (synovial membrane)	it is a connective tissue membrane that covers the inner surface of joint capsule. When the synovium is inflamed, the term of synovitis is used
Sub-acromial place	acromion is a bony process in upper outer of the scapula
Dextrose prolotherapy	local injection of dextrose works as an irritant and provokes the body immune system to relive the inflammation

Author details

Mohammad Ahmadi-Dastgerdi[1*], Nafiseh Bavaghar[2] and Aniseh Bavaghar[3]

1 Shahid Beheshti University of Medical Science, Tehran, Iran

2 Iran University of Medical Science, Tehran, Iran

3 Tehran University of Medical Science, Tehran, Iran

*Address all correspondence to: mo.ahmadi1370@gmail.com

References

[1] Yu KH, Chen HH, Cheng TT, Jan YJ, Weng MY, Lin YJ, et al. Consensus recommendations on managing the selected comorbidities including cardiovascular disease, osteoporosis, and interstitial lung disease in rheumatoid arthritis. Medicine (Baltimore). 2022;**101**(1):e28501. DOI: 10.1097/MD.0000000000028501

[2] Rice JB, White AG, Scarpati LM, Wan G, Nelson WW. Long-term systemic corticosteroid exposure: A systematic literature review. Clinical Therapeutics. 2017;**39**(11):2216-2229. DOI: 10.1016/j.clinthera.2017.09.011

[3] Rayegani SM, Raeissadat SA, Ahmadi-Dastgerdi M, Bavaghar N, Rahimi-Dehgolan S. Comparing the efficacy of local triamcinolone injection in carpal tunnel syndrome using three different approaches with or without ultrasound guidance. Journal of Pain Research. 2019;**12**:2951-2958. DOI: 10.2147/JPR.S212948

[4] Salman Roghani R, Holisaz MT, Tarkashvand M. et al., Different doses of steroid injection in elderly patients with carpal tunnel syndrome: A triple-blind, randomized, controlled trial. Clinical Intervention Aging. 2018;**13**:117-124. DOI: 10.2147/CIA.S151290

[5] Phillips M, Bhandari M, Grant J, Bedi A, Trojian T, Johnson A, et al. A systematic review of current clinical practice guidelines on intra-articular hyaluronic acid, corticosteroid, and platelet-rich plasma injection for knee osteoarthritis: An international perspective. Orthopaedic Journal of Sports Medicine. 2021;**9**(8):2325. DOI: 10.1177/23259671211030272

[6] Keidan T, Saleh S, Svorai Band S, Gannot G, Oron A. Clinical presentation and treatment. Harefuah. 2022;**161**(11):706-708

[7] Brun SP. Idiopathic frozen shoulder. Australia Journal of Genetic Practice. 2019;**48**(11):757-761. DOI: 10.31128/AJGP-07-19-4992

[8] Koh KH. Corticosteroid injection for adhesive capsulitis in primary care: A systematic review of randomised clinical trials. Singapore Medical Journal. 2016;**57**(12):646-657. DOI: 10.11622/smedj.2016146

[9] Bayat M, Raeissadat SA, Mortazavian Babaki M, Rahimi-Dehgolan S. Is dextrose prolotherapy superior to corticosteroid injection In patients with chronic lateral epicondylitis?: A randomized clinical trial. Orthopedic Research and Reviews. 2019;**11**:167-175. DOI: 10.2147/ORR.S218698

[10] Foster ZJ, Voss TT, Hatch J, Frimodig A. Corticosteroid injections for common musculoskeletal conditions. American Family Physician. 2015;**92**(8):694-699

[11] Seigerman D, McEntee RM, Matzon J, Lutsky K, Fletcher D, Rivlin M, et al. Time to improvement after corticosteroid injection for trigger finger. Cureus. 2021;**13**(8):e16856. DOI: 10.7759/cureus.16856

[12] Pianka MA, Serino J, DeFroda SF, Bodendorfer BM. Greater trochanteric pain syndrome: Evaluation and management of a wide spectrum of pathology. SAGE Open Medicine. 2021;**9**:2050. DOI: 10.1177/2050312 1211022582

[13] Raeissadat SA, Ghazi Hosseini P, Bahrami MH, Salman

Roghani R, Fathi M, Gharooee Ahangar A, et al. The comparison effects of intra-articular injection of platelet rich plasma (PRP), plasma rich in growth factor (PRGF), hyaluronic acid (HA), and ozone in knee osteoarthritis; a one year randomized clinical trial. BMC Musculoskeletal Disorders. 2021;**22**(1):134. DOI: 10.1186/s12891-021-04017-x

[14] Vaienti E, Scita G, Ceccarelli F, Pogliacomi F. Understanding the human knee and its relationship to total knee replacement. Acta Bio-Medica. 2017;**88**(2S):6-16. DOI: 10.23750/abm.v88i2-S.6507

[15] Wu T, Zhao WH, Dong Y, Song HX, Li JH. Effectiveness of ultrasound-guided versus fluoroscopy or computed tomography scanning guidance in lumbar facet joint injections in adults with facet joint syndrome: A meta-analysis of controlled trials. Archives of Physical Medicine and Rehabilitation. 2016;**97**(9):1558-1563. DOI: 10.1016/j.apmr.2015.11.013

[16] Bodor M, Murthy N, Uribe Y. Ultrasound-guided cervical facet joint injections. The Spine Journal. 2022;**22**(6):983-992. DOI: 10.1016/j.spinee.2022.01.011

[17] Manchikanti L, Candido KD, Kaye AD, Boswell MV, Benyamin RM, Falco FJ, et al. Randomized trial of epidural injections for spinal stenosis published in the New England Journal of Medicine: Further confusion without clarification. Pain Physician. 2014;**17**(4):E475-E488

Chapter 3

Inhaled Corticosteroids: Benefits and Risks

Hanaa Shafiek

Abstract

Airway diseases, mainly asthma and chronic obstructive pulmonary diseases (COPD), are frequently treated with inhaled corticosteroids (ICS). ICS are considered as the cornerstone of asthma management, however, in COPD the picture is different and ICS are indicated in special circumstances. The benefits of ICS are well documented in controlling disease symptomatology. But, still there are side effects of using ICS, especially the risk of pneumonia and bacterial colonization of the airways. In this chapter, I will explore the change in the use of ICS in asthma and COPD, the indications of ICS, the benefits of ICS and its drawbacks, and how we could modify our practice in order to avoid the side effects of ICS.

Keywords: airway inflammation, asthma, chronic obstructive pulmonary disease, inhaled corticosteroids types, complications

1. Introduction

Systemic Corticosteroids (SC) are synthetic analogs of the naturally occurring steroid hormones produced by the cortex of the adrenal gland that is administrated by oral or injectable routes. The SC hormones have glucocorticoid and mineralocorticoid properties with varying degrees. The most important is the glucocorticoids which are predominantly involved in metabolism and have immunosuppressive, anti-inflammatory, and vasoconstrictive effects. SC is widely prescribed in medicine including respiratory medicine as in airway diseases, sarcoidosis, interstitial lung diseases, pulmonary eosinophilic diseases and others [1]. Since the 1950s, SC has been proven to be an effective therapy for persistent asthma [2, 3], however, they have various side effects.

The first pressurized metered-dose inhaler (pMDI) as a bronchodilator for asthma, was introduced in 1956 namely non-selective beta-2-agonists isoprenaline and adrenaline that was associated with rapid relief of asthma symptoms [4]. In the 1960s, there was an epidemic of asthma deaths in Britain thought to be caused by the high use of inhaled bronchodilators [5, 6] and so delayed in seeking medical advice, even if not proved, resulted in suspending the use of inhaled isoprenaline that was replaced later by salbutamol, the selective short-acting beta-2-agonist, and increase the use of SC [4]. By the early 1970s, inhaled beclomethasone dipropionate started to develop as 1st inhaled corticosteroid (ICS) and placebo-controlled studies confirmed

IntechOpen

the value of ICS therapy in asthma [7–9]. Afterward, ICS became the cornerstone of asthma management and various substitutes and forms were introduced in pulmonary medicine.

2. Mechanisms of ICS

ICS have glucocorticoids effects that suppress the ongoing inflammatory process through gene transcription mechanisms [10, 11]. Glucocorticoids act by binding to glucocorticoid receptors (GRs) in the cytoplasm resulting in their activation and translocation in the nucleus to produce their anti-inflammatory effects through various molecular effects.

Corticosteroids switch off various activated inflammatory genes that encode cytokines, chemokines, inflammatory enzymes and proteins as the anti-inflammatory proteins secretory leukoprotease inhibitor, and mitogen-activated protein kinase phosphatase-1 (MKP-1) which inhibits MAP kinase pathways [12, 13]. The nuclear GR interacts with coactivator molecules as CREB-binding protein resulting in the activation of proinflammatory transcription factors, nuclear factor-κB (NF-κB) and activator protein-1, in the airways and so reduces histone acetyltransferase activity [10, 14]. Also, activated GR recruits histone deacetylase-2 (HDAC2) to the activated inflammatory gene complex which reverses histone acetylation resulting in the suppression of all nuclear-activated inflammatory genes [15].

Further, ICS increase the gene transcription encoding β_2-receptors, resulting in increased expression of β_2-receptors on the cell surface of the airways [16, 17] which protect against the β_2-receptors tolerance after long-term use. Moreover, ICS may enhance the β_2-receptors coupling to G-proteins that promote β_2-agonist effects and reverse its uncoupling in response to some inflammatory mediators as interleukin-1β through G-protein coupled receptor kinase stimulation [18]. β_2-Agonists also increase the translocation of GR to the nucleus after its activation thus enhancing corticosteroids' anti-inflammatory effects through synchronized interactions [19, 20].

On the other hand, ICS have cellular effects by reducing the numbers of various inflammatory cells mainly eosinophils, mast cell, T-lymphocytes and dendritic cells through either inhibiting the recruitment of these cells in the airways or their survival [21]. Moreover, ICS restore the airway epithelial cell integrity thus inhibiting the transcription of inflammatory genes thus suppressing mucosal inflammation and eosinophilic recruitment into the airways that is associated with airway hyperreactivity [22, 23].

3. Types of ICS

Nowadays, there are eight different ICS molecules available. These are: beclomethasone dipropionate (BMD) which is the first known ICS, budesonide (BUD), ciclesonide (CC), flunisolide, fluticasone propionate (FP), fluticasone furoate (FF), triamcinolone acetonide (TA) and mometasone furoate (MF). The difference between these molecules is lipophilia with greater GR affinity and longer duration of action; as fluticasone furoate is the most lipophilic (i.e., high potency) and beclomethasone dipropionate the lowest [24].

DOI: http://dx.doi.org/10.5772/intechopen.110753

The various ICS have also different pulmonary bioavailability (i.e., within the airways) and oral bioavailability (i.e., in the systemic circulation) [25]. Negligible oral bioavailability due to high first-pass metabolism is found for FF, FP, MF and CC and so fewer side effects [24]. Three factors are expected to affect the efficacy of an ICS: the potency (the lower inhaled dose occupied the same number of GRs), the delivered dose (the device efficiency) and airway residency duration. FF, FP, MF and CC have greater residency duration in the airways which allows one daily dose; however, twice daily is considered better [26, 27]. **Figure 1** shows the relationship between ICS dose and its affinity to GR, whereas FF has both the higher GR affinity with the lowest dose compared to triamcinolone acetonide and flunisolide [28].

ICS could be delivered by pressurized metered-dose (pMDI) inhaler, dry-powder (DPI) inhaler and nebulization which are expected to influence the ICS dose. The great difference between the devices is the size of respirable particles emitted that are generally <5 μm [29]. DPI and pMDI (with drugs dissolved in chlorofluorocarbon "CFC") usually emit particles between 3 and 5 μm, however, pMDI with drugs dissolved in hydrofluoroalkane (HFA) emits ultrafine particles of about 1 μm which allow high delivery of ICS in low-mid doses with high lung deposition. **Table 1** compares the low-, mid- and high-doses of ICS of different molecules and devices. Regarding fluticasone, according to the manufacturer's summary of Product Characteristics, FF 100 μg once daily is approximately equivalent to FP 250 μg twice daily [35]. The devices nowadays are many, especially those designed to deliver the DPI either pre-metered or device-metered (**Figure 2**) [36].

In addition, the GINA guidelines has published equivalent doses of different ICS molecules (**Table 2**) [37].

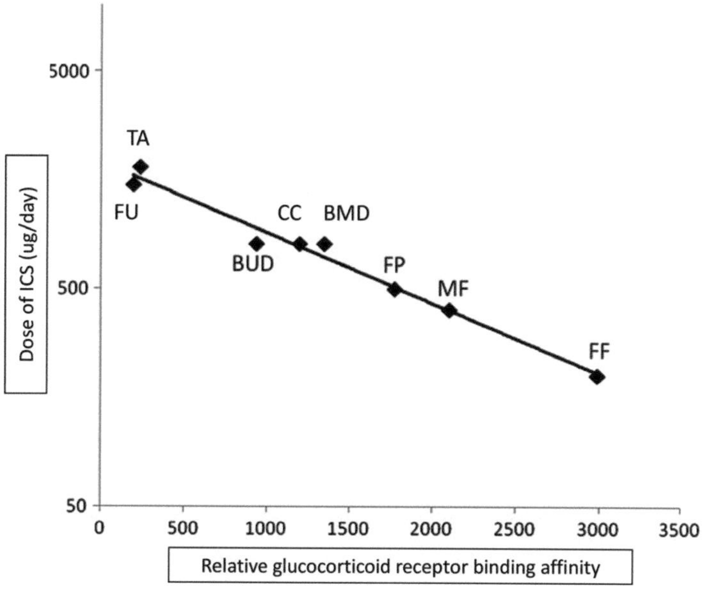

Figure 1.
Relationship between the dose of ICS and relative glucocorticoid receptor binding affinity [28].

ICS molecule	Age	Low-dose	Mid-dose	High-dose
Beclomethasone HFA/pMDI	0–4 years	NA	NA	NA
	5–11 years	80–160 µg	160–320 µg	>320 µg
	≥12 years	80–240 µg	240–480 µg	>480 µg
Budesonide DPI	0–4 years	NA	NA	NA
	5–11 years	180–400 µg	400–800 µg	>800 µg
	≥12 years	180–600 µg	600–1200 µg	>1200 µg
Fluticasone HFA/pMDI	0–4 years	176 µg	176–352 µg	352 µg
	5–11 years	88–176 µg	176–352 µg	>352 µg
	≥12 years	88–264 µg	264–440 µg	>440 µg
Fluticasone DPI	0–4 years	NA	NA	NA
	5–11 years	100–200 µg	200–400 µg	>400 µg
	≥12 years	100–300 µg	300–500 µg	>500 µg
Mometasone DPI	0–4 years	NA	NA	NA
	5–11 years	NA	NA	NA
	≥12 years	200 µg	400 µg	>400 µg
Budesonide nebulized (solution inhalation)	0–4 years	0.25–0.5 mg	0.5–1 mg	>1 mg
	5–11 years	0.5 mg	1 mg	2 mg
	≥12 years	NA	NA	NA

**All doses are per day.*

Table 1.
Comparison between ICS molecules classified by doses [30–34].*

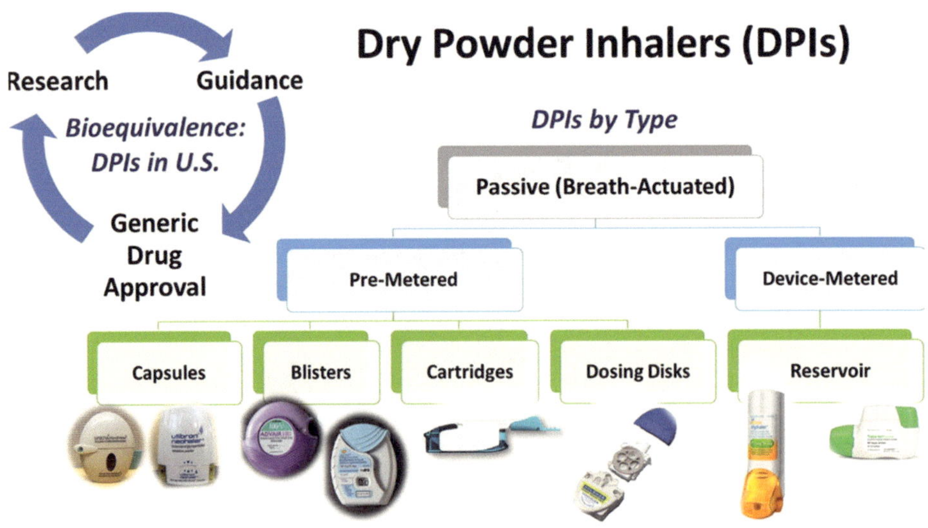

Figure 2.
Classifications of drug powder inhalers (DPI) [36].

ICS molecule	Age	Low-dose	Mid-dose	High-dose
Beclomethasone HFA/ pMDI	5–11 years	100–200 µg	>200–400 µg	> 400 µg
	≥12 years	200–500 µg	> 500–1000 µg	>1000 µg
Budesonide (DPI, pMDI, standard particle or HFA)	5–11 years	50–100 µg	>100–200 µg	>200 µg
	≥12 years	200–400 µg	>400–800 µg	>800 µg
Fluticasone furoate DPI	5–11 years	50 µg		NA
	≥12 years	100 µg		200 µg
Fluticasone propionate (DPI, pMDI, standard particle or HFA)	5–11 years	50–100 µg	100–200 µg	>200 µg
	≥12 years	100–250 µg	250–500 µg	>500 µg
Mometasone (pMDI, standard particle or HFA)	5–11 years	100	200	5–11 years
	≥12 years	200–400 µg		>400 µg
Ciclosonide pMDI /HFA	5–11 years	80	>80–160	>160
	≥12 years	80–160	>160–320	>320

Table 2.
Comparison between ICS molecules classified by doses as published in GINA guidelines.

4. Clinical uses and benefits of ICS

4.1 Asthma

ICS are considered as the cornerstone treatment for the management of asthma in all ages. ICS are the first line of therapy for persistent asthma with a starting low-dose that to be increased according to the level of control of the disease including the addition of other types of inhalers such as long-acting- β_2-agonist (LABA) and/or long-acting muscarinic antagonists (LAMA) in a step-wise approach [37]. In addition, in the latest GINA guidelines [37], low-dose ICS in combination with formoterol (a LABA inhaler) was approved as a reliever instead of short-acting β_2-agonist (SABA) as salbutamol that was associated with a decrease risk of severe exacerbations and is called the anti-inflammatory reliever.

Moreover, it is recommended the addition of low-dose ICS in the management of mild asthma. Juniper et al. showed that the use of low-dose ICS in mild asthma was associated with less symptoms and improvement of lung function up to being asymptomatic over several months of therapy [38]. Further, Pauwels et al. reported a reduction in asthma exacerbations among mild asthmatics treated with low-dose ICS [39]. Recent GINA guidelines recommend the use of low-dose ICS or low-dose ICS-formoterol as a reliever for mild asthma to decrease the risk of severe asthma exacerbation based on various studies [40–42]. Medium to high dose ICS are recommended for persistent asthma according to the step-wise approach of GINA guidelines [37]. ICS are also related to improvement in lung function in asthmatic children and adults [43, 44] owing to the switch-off of the chronic inflammatory process by ICS in asthma. Further, many studies showed that regular ICS use provides significant protection and reduces the risk of mortality, severe exacerbation and hospitalization of asthma population [39, 45, 46].

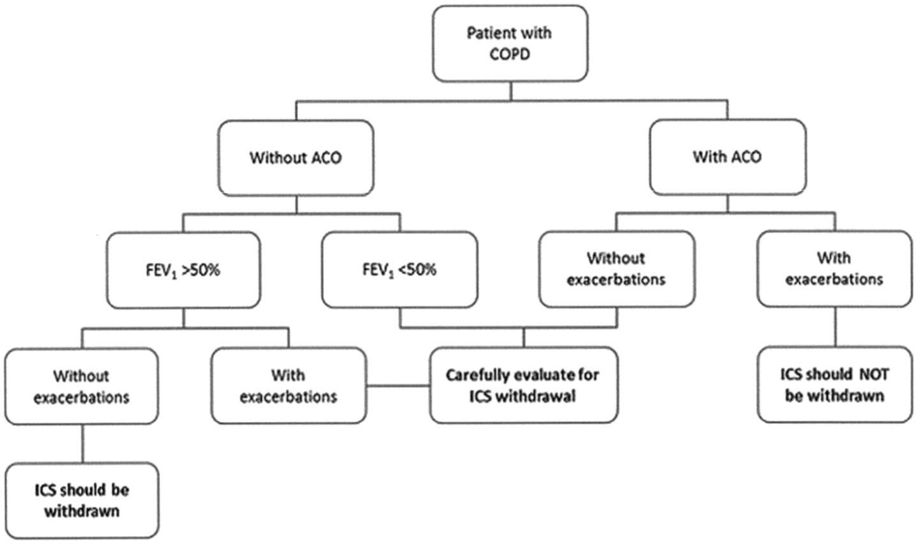

Figure 3.
Algorithm for ICS withdrawal in COPD [54].

4.2 Chronic obstructive pulmonary disease (COPD)

The use of ICS is controversial in COPD medications. The response to ICS in COPD patients is less than asthma population [47] which reflects the resistance of airway inflammation to ICS secondary to the reduction of HDAC2 [48, 49]. According to Global Initiative Lung Disease (GOLD) guidelines of COPD [50], ICS are indicated in frequent COPD exacerbator phenotype (i.e., those who had ≥2 exacerbations/year required OCS or ≥ 1 exacerbation need hospitalization) or COPD patients with blood eosinophilia ≥300 cells/μL [51]. Also, the Spanish guidelines of COPD, recommended the use of ICS in asthma-COPD overlap (ACO) who are patients with criteria of asthma and COPD with blood eosinophil counts >300 cells/μL and/or a post-bronchodilator response of >400 mL and 15% in FEV_1 [52]. A meta-analysis of important studies in COPD reported that ICS withdrawal did not result in a significant increase in COPD exacerbations risk [53]. Miravitlles et al. proposed an algorithm for the withdrawal of ICS in COPD patients based on FEV_1% predicted and exacerbation history [54]. **Figure 3** summarizes this algorithm [54].

5. Risks and complications of ICS

5.1 Local effects

ICS are associated with some local side effects, despite being not serious but could be associated with discontinuation of therapy. Hoarseness of the voice or dysphonia is the most common local side effect that occurs in about 50% of ICS users. It is a reversible side effect of drug withdrawal that is attributed to myopathy of laryngeal muscles [55]. Oropharyngeal candidiasis is the second most common side effect, despite being more in the elderly population, a percentage of ICS users complaint of it which is related to poor inhalation technique and high doses of ICS. The use of spacers is associated with decreasing these side effects [37, 56].

Importantly, ICS are associated with an increased risk of pneumonia. Patients with COPD, older patients, active smokers, low body mass index <25 kg/m^2, patients with a history of exacerbations or pneumonia, and/or severe airflow limitation are associated with a higher risk of pneumonia on ICS use [57, 58]. In a meta-analysis, both inhaled fluticasone and budesonide were associated with a significant risk of pneumonia [59] that could be related to the use of a high dose of ICS alone or in-combination with bronchodilator [60]. Further, ICS use was associated with a specific bacterial infection in a subset of the severe COPD population. Shafiek et al. [61] found that ICS dose could be associated with *Pseudomonas aeruginosa* infection in the severe COPD population. This could be explained on the basis of impaired recognition of *P. aeruginosa* and activity of alveolar macrophages secondary to altered expression of Toll-like receptor 2 and various cytokine production in COPD patients receiving ICS [62]. On the other hand, O'Byrne et al. found that budesonide, as an ICS, was not associated with increased risk of pneumonia in asthmatic patients [63]. However, Qian et al. found that ICS use is associated with increased risk of pneumonia in asthma population with a risk of 1.44/1000 asthmatics/year [64].

A recent meta-analysis showed that ICS in high doses of fluticasone is associated with an increased risk of non-tuberculous mycobacteria in chronic respiratory diseases, and also may be associated with tuberculosis, especially in COPD patients [65].

5.2 Systemic effects

The use of ICS is less associated with systemic side effects compared to OCS. However, long-term ICS use is associated with an increased risk of bone fractures in patients with COPD which was reported to be up to 27% in a meta-analysis of various RCTs and observational studies with fluticasone or budesonide therapy [66]. Although bone density is less in patients taking high-dose of ICS, interpretation is confounded by the fact that these patients are also taking intermittent courses of OCS [21]. Further, osteoporosis is strongly correlated to COPD due to various lifestyle risk factors such as poor physical inactivity and smoking, vitamin D deficiency and COPD-associated inflammation [67].

Hypothalamic–pituitary–adrenal axis suppression is associated mainly with OCS for weeks even with short courses, but with ICS the results of the studies are inconsistent as often the patients have also been taking courses of OCS [68]. Increased risk of new-onset diabetes or diabetes progression has been reported in ICS users which was about 34% and is more among high doses ICS users and COPD [69]. Further, cataracts [70] and glaucoma [71] have been reported as side effects of high doses of ICS.

6. Conclusions

The introduction of ICS in respiratory medicine is crucial and modifies the management of diseases. ICS are good anti-inflammatory medication. ICS can effectively replace OCS in the control of chronic obstructive respiratory diseases, especially asthma. However, ICS has still side effects, especially in high doses; despite being less than OCS, it is associated with some morbidity that should be well controlled and managed.

Conflict of interest

I declare that I have no conflicts in relation to the current work.

Author details

Hanaa Shafiek
Alexandria Faculty of Medicine, Alexandria University, Alexandria, Egypt

*Address all correspondence to: whitecoat.med@gmail.com

References

[1] Sethi GR, Singhal KK. Pulmonary diseases and corticosteroids. Indian Journal of Pediatrics. 2008;**75**(10):1045-1056. Epub 2008/11/22. DOI: 10.1007/s12098-008-0209-0

[2] Carryer HM, Koelsche GA, Prickman LE, Maytum CK, Lake CF, Williams HL. The effect of cortisone of bronchial asthma and hay fever occurring in subjects sensitive to ragweed pollen. The Journal of Allergy. 1950;**21**(4):282-287. Epub 1950/07/01. DOI: 10.1016/0021-8707(50)90059-1

[3] CONTROLLED trial of effects of cortisone acetate in chronic asthma; report to the Medical Research Council by the subcommittee on clinical trials in asthma. Lancet. 1956;**271**(6947):798-803. Epub 1956/10/20

[4] Crompton G. A brief history of inhaled asthma therapy over the last fifty years. Primary Care Respiratory Journal. 2006;**15**(6):326-331. Epub 2006/11/10. DOI: 10.1016/j.pcrj.2006.09.002

[5] Speizer FE, Doll R, Heaf P, Strang LB. Investigation into use of drugs preceding death from asthma. British Medical Journal. 1968;**1**(5588):339-343. Epub 1968/02/10. DOI: 10.1136/bmj.1.5588.339

[6] Inman WH, Adelstein AM. Rise and fall of asthma mortality in England and Wales in relation to use of pressurised aerosols. Lancet. 1969;**2**(7615):279-285. Epub 1969/08/09. DOI: 10.1016/s0140-6736(69)90051-8

[7] Cameron SJ, Cooper EJ, Crompton GK, Hoare MV, Grant IW. Substitution of beclomethasone aerosol for oral prednisolone in the treatment of chronic asthma. British Medical Journal. 1973;**4**(5886):205-207. Epub 1973/10/27. DOI: 10.1136/bmj.4.5886.205

[8] Hodson ME, Batten JC, Clarke SW, Gregg I. Beclomethasone dipropionate aerosol in asthma. Transfer of steroid-dependent asthmatic patients from oral prednisone to beclomethasone dipropionate aerosol. The American Review of Respiratory Disease. 1974;**110**(4):403-408. Epub 1974/10/01. DOI: 10.1164/arrd.1974.110.4.403

[9] Vilsvik JS, Schaanning J. Beclomethasone dipropionate aerosol in adult steroid-dependent obstructive lung disease. Scandinavian Journal of Respiratory Diseases. 1974;**55**(3):169-175 Epub 1974/01/01

[10] Barnes PJ. How corticosteroids control inflammation: Quintiles prize lecture 2005. British Journal of Pharmacology. 2006;**148**(3):245-254. Epub 2006/04/11. DOI: 10.1038/sj.bjp.0706736

[11] Rhen T, Cidlowski JA. Antiinflammatory action of glucocorticoids--new mechanisms for old drugs. The New England Journal of Medicine. 2005;**353**(16):1711-1723. Epub 2005/10/21. DOI: 10.1056/NEJMra050541

[12] Clark AR, Martins JR, Tchen CR. Role of dual specificity phosphatases in biological responses to glucocorticoids. The Journal of Biological Chemistry. 2008;**283**(38):25765-25769. Epub 2008/06/11. DOI: 10.1074/jbc.R700053200

[13] Barnes PJ. Corticosteroid effects on cell signalling. The European Respiratory Journal. 2006;**27**(2):413-426. Epub 2006/02/03. DOI: 10.1183/09031936.06.00125404

[14] Barnes PJ, Adcock IM, Ito K. Histone acetylation and deacetylation: Importance in inflammatory lung diseases. The European Respiratory Journal. 2005;**25**(3):552-563. Epub 2005/03/02. DOI: 10.1183/09031936.05.00117504

[15] Ito K, Barnes PJ, Adcock IM. Glucocorticoid receptor recruitment of histone deacetylase 2 inhibits interleukin-1beta-induced histone H4 acetylation on lysines 8 and 12. Molecular and Cellular Biology. 2000;**20**(18):6891-6903. Epub 2000/08/25. DOI: 10.1128/mcb.20.18.6891-6903.2000

[16] Mak JC, Nishikawa M, Barnes PJ. Glucocorticosteroids increase beta 2-adrenergic receptor transcription in human lung. The American Journal of Physiology. 1995;**268**(1 Pt 1):L41-L46. Epub 1995/01/01. DOI: 10.1152/ajplung.1995.268.1.L41

[17] Baraniuk JN, Ali M, Brody D, Maniscalco J, Gaumond E, Fitzgerald T, et al. Glucocorticoids induce beta2-adrenergic receptor function in human nasal mucosa. American Journal of Respiratory and Critical Care Medicine. 1997;**155**(2):704-710. Epub 1997/02/01. DOI: 10.1164/ajrccm.155.2.9032216

[18] Mak JC, Chuang TT, Harris CA, Barnes PJ. Increased expression of G protein-coupled receptor kinases in cystic fibrosis lung. European Journal of Pharmacology. 2002;**436**(3):165-172. Epub 2002/02/23. DOI: 10.1016/s0014-2999(01)01625-9

[19] Usmani OS, Ito K, Maneechotesuwan K, Ito M, Johnson M, Barnes PJ, et al. Glucocorticoid receptor nuclear translocation in airway cells after inhaled combination therapy. American Journal of Respiratory and Critical Care Medicine. 2005;**172**(6):704-712. Epub 2005/04/30. DOI: 10.1164/rccm.200408-1041OC

[20] Roth M, Johnson PR, Rüdiger JJ, King GG, Ge Q, Burgess JK, et al. Interaction between glucocorticoids and beta2 agonists on bronchial airway smooth muscle cells through synchronised cellular signalling. Lancet. 2002;**360**(9342):1293-1299. Epub 2002/11/05. DOI: 10.1016/s0140-6736(02)11319-5

[21] Barnes PJ. Inhaled corticosteroids. Pharmaceuticals (Basel). 2010;**3**(3):514-540. Epub 2010/03/08. DOI: 10.3390/ph3030514

[22] Ketchell RI, Jensen MW, Lumley P, Wright AM, Allenby MI, O'Connor BJ. Rapid effect of inhaled fluticasone propionate on airway responsiveness to adenosine 5′-monophosphate in mild asthma. The Journal of Allergy and Clinical Immunology. 2002;**110**(4):603-606. Epub 2002/10/10. DOI: 10.1067/mai.2002.128486

[23] Erin EM, Zacharasiewicz AS, Nicholson GC, Tan AJ, Neighbour H, Engelstätter R, et al. Rapid effect of inhaled ciclesonide in asthma: A randomized, placebo-controlled study. Chest. 2008;**134**(4):740-745. Epub 2008/04/12. DOI: 10.1378/chest.07-2575

[24] Daley-Yates PT. Inhaled corticosteroids: Potency, dose equivalence and therapeutic index. British Journal of Clinical Pharmacology. 2015;**80**(3):372-380. Epub 2015/03/27. DOI: 10.1111/bcp.12637

[25] Duse M, Santamaria F, Verga MC, Bergamini M, Simeone G, Leonardi L, et al. Inter-society consensus for the use of inhaled corticosteroids in infants, children and adolescents with airway diseases. Italian Journal of Pediatrics. 2021;**47**(1):97. DOI: 10.1186/s13052-021-01013-8

[26] Woodcock A, Bleecker ER, Busse WW, Lötvall J, Snowise NG,

Frith L, et al. Fluticasone furoate: Once-daily evening treatment versus twice-daily treatment in moderate asthma. Respiratory Research. 2011;**12**(1):160. Epub 2011/12/23. DOI: 10.1186/1465-9921-12-160

[27] Boulet LP, Cowie RL, Negro RD, Brett W, Gold M, Marques A, et al. Comparison of once- with twice-daily dosing of fluticasone propionate in mild and moderate asthma. Canadian Respiratory Journal. 2000;**7**(3):239-247. Epub 2000/07/21. DOI: 10.1155/2000/464639

[28] Electronic Medicines Compendium. Datapharm Communications Limited AahwmouelaM

[29] Daley-Yates P, editor Relationship between pharmacokinetic and aerodynamic particle size distribution properties for inhalers containing corticosteroids. Respiratory Drug Delivery; 2014

[30] Liu T, Han M, Tian F, Cun D, Rantanen J, Yang M. Budesonide nanocrystal-loaded hyaluronic acid microparticles for inhalation: In vitro and in vivo evaluation. Carbohydrate Polymers. 2018;**181**:1143-1152. Epub 2017/12/20. DOI: 10.1016/j.carbpol.2017.11.018

[31] Miyazaki Y, Aruga N, Kadota K, Tozuka Y, Takeuchi H. Improved respirable fraction of budesonide powder for dry powder inhaler formulations produced by advanced supercritical CO(2) processing and use of a novel additive. International Journal of Pharmaceutics. 2017;**528**(1-2):118-126. Epub 2017/06/07. DOI: 10.1016/j.ijpharm.2017.06.002

[32] Kobayashi Y, Asako M, Yamamoto T, Yasuba H, Tomoda K, Kanda A. Replacement of SFC-DPI with SFC-MDI exhaled through the nose improves eosinophilic chronic rhinosinusitis in patients with bronchial asthma. International Journal of Clinical Pharmacology and Therapeutics. 2017;**55**(1):89-94. Epub 2016/11/24. DOI: 10.5414/cp202633

[33] Sher LD, Yiu G, Sakov A, Liu S, Caracta CF. Fluticasone propionate and fluticasone propionate/salmeterol multidose dry powder inhalers compared with placebo for persistent asthma. Allergy and Asthma Proceedings. 2017;**38**(5):343-353. Epub 2017/06/24. DOI: 10.2500/aap.2017.38.4069

[34] Cloutier MM, Baptist AP, Blake KV, Brooks EG, Bryant-Stephens T, DiMango E, et al. 2020 focused updates to the asthma management guidelines: A report from the National Asthma Education and prevention program coordinating committee expert panel working group. The Journal of Allergy and Clinical Immunology. 2020;**146**(6):1217-1270. Epub 2020/12/08. DOI: 10.1016/j.jaci.2020.10.003

[35] Available from: https://northeast.devonformularyguidance.nhs.uk/formulary/chapters/3.-respiratory/corticosteroid-inhaler-preparations-equivalent-beclometasone-bdp.

[36] Newman B, Babiskin A, Bielski E, Boc S, Dhapare S, Fang L, et al. Scientific and regulatory activities initiated by the U.S. food and drug administration to foster approvals of generic dry powder inhalers: Bioequivalence perspective. Advanced Drug Delivery Reviews. 2022;**190**:114526. DOI: 10.1016/j.addr.2022.114526

[37] Global initiative for asthma. Global Strategy for Asthma Management and Prevention AN, 1, 2021. Available from: https://ginasthma.org/wp-content/

uploads/2021/05/GINA-Main-Report-2021-V2-WMS.pdf.

[38] Juniper EF, Kline PA, Vanzieleghem MA, Ramsdale EH, O'Byrne PM, Hargreave FE. Effect of long-term treatment with an inhaled corticosteroid (budesonide) on airway hyperresponsiveness and clinical asthma in nonsteroid-dependent asthmatics. The American Review of Respiratory Disease. 1990;**142**(4):832-836. Epub 1990/10/01. DOI: 10.1164/ajrccm/142.4.832

[39] Pauwels RA, Pedersen S, Busse WW, Tan WC, Chen YZ, Ohlsson SV, et al. Early intervention with budesonide in mild persistent asthma: A randomised, double-blind trial. Lancet. 2003;**361**(9363):1071-1076. Epub 2003/04/04. DOI: 10.1016/s0140-6736(03)12891-7

[40] O'Byrne PM, FitzGerald JM, Bateman ED, Barnes PJ, Zhong N, Keen C, et al. Inhaled combined budesonide-Formoterol as needed in mild asthma. The New England Journal of Medicine. 2018;**378**(20):1865-1876. Epub 2018/05/17. DOI: 10.1056/NEJMoa1715274

[41] Bateman ED, Reddel HK, O'Byrne PM, Barnes PJ, Zhong N, Keen C, et al. As-needed budesonide-Formoterol versus maintenance budesonide in mild asthma. The New England Journal of Medicine. 2018;**378**(20):1877-1887. Epub 2018/05/17. DOI: 10.1056/NEJMoa1715275

[42] Hardy J, Baggott C, Fingleton J, Reddel HK, Hancox RJ, Harwood M, et al. Budesonide-formoterol reliever therapy versus maintenance budesonide plus terbutaline reliever therapy in adults with mild to moderate asthma (PRACTICAL): A 52-week, open-label, multicentre, superiority, randomised controlled trial. Lancet. 2019;**394**(10202):919-928. Epub 2019/08/28. DOI: 10.1016/s0140-6736(19)31948-8

[43] Agertoft L, Pedersen S. Effects of long-term treatment with an inhaled corticosteroid on growth and pulmonary function in asthmatic children. Respiratory Medicine. 1994;**88**(5):373-381. Epub 1994/05/01. DOI: 10.1016/0954-6111(94)90044-2

[44] Selroos O, Pietinalho A, Löfroos AB, Riska H. Effect of early vs late intervention with inhaled corticosteroids in asthma. Chest. 1995;**108**(5):1228-1234. Epub 1995/11/01. DOI: 10.1378/chest.108.5.1228

[45] Suissa S, Ernst P, Benayoun S, Baltzan M, Cai B. Low-dose inhaled corticosteroids and the prevention of death from asthma. The New England Journal of Medicine. 2000;**343**(5):332-336. Epub 2000/08/03. DOI: 10.1056/nejm200008033430504

[46] O'Byrne PM, Barnes PJ, Rodriguez-Roisin R, Runnerstrom E, Sandstrom T, Svensson K, et al. Low dose inhaled budesonide and formoterol in mild persistent asthma: The OPTIMA randomized trial. American Journal of Respiratory and Critical Care Medicine. 2001;**164**(8 Pt 1):1392-1397. Epub 2001/11/13. DOI: 10.1164/ajrccm.164.8.2104102

[47] Suissa S, Barnes PJ. Inhaled corticosteroids in COPD: The case against. The European Respiratory Journal. 2009;**34**(1):13-16. Epub 2009/07/02. DOI: 10.1183/09031936.00190908

[48] Barnes PJ. Role of HDAC2 in the pathophysiology of COPD. Annual Review of Physiology. 2009;**71**:451-464. Epub 2008/09/27. DOI: 10.1146/annurev.physiol.010908.163257

[49] Adcock IM, Cosio B, Tsaprouni L, Barnes PJ, Ito K. Redox regulation of histone deacetylases and glucocorticoid-mediated inhibition of the inflammatory response. Antioxidants & Redox Signaling. 2005;7(1-2):144-152. Epub 2005/01/15. DOI: 10.1089/ars.2005.7.144

[50] The Global Initiative for Chronic Obstructive Lung Disease (GOLD). The 2023 global strategy for the diagnosis m, and prevention of chronic obstructive pulmonary disease (COPD). Available at: https://goldcopd.org/2023-gold-report-2/.

[51] Venkatesan P. GOLD COPD report: 2023 update. The Lancet Respiratory Medicine. 2023;**11**(1):18. Epub 2022/12/04. DOI: 10.1016/S2213-2600(22)00494-5

[52] Miravitlles M, Alvarez-Gutierrez FJ, Calle M, Casanova C, Cosio BG, López-Viña A, et al. Algorithm for identification of asthma-COPD overlap: consensus between the Spanish COPD and asthma guidelines. Eur Respir J. 2017;**49**(5). Epub 2017/05/04. DOI: 10.1183/13993003.00068-2017

[53] Nadeem NJ, Taylor SJ, Eldridge SM. Withdrawal of inhaled corticosteroids in individuals with COPD--a systematic review and comment on trial methodology. Respiratory Research. 2011;**12**(1):107. Epub 2011/08/16. DOI: 10.1186/1465-9921-12-107

[54] Miravitlles M, Cosío BG, Arnedillo A, Calle M, Alcázar-Navarrete B, González C, et al. A proposal for the withdrawal of inhaled corticosteroids in the clinical practice of chronic obstructive pulmonary disease. Respiratory Research. 2017;**18**(1):198. Epub 2017/12/01. DOI: 10.1186/s12931-017-0682-y

[55] Williamson IJ, Matusiewicz SP, Brown PH, Greening AP, Crompton GK. Frequency of voice problems and cough in patients using pressurized aerosol inhaled steroid preparations. The European Respiratory Journal. 1995;**8**(4):590-592 Epub 1995/04/01

[56] Toogood JH, Jennings B, Greenway RW, Chuang L. Candidiasis and dysphonia complicating beclomethasone treatment of asthma. The Journal of Allergy and Clinical Immunology. 1980;**65**(2):145-153. Epub 1980/02/01. DOI: 10.1016/0091-6749(80)90200-6

[57] Vogelmeier CF, Criner GJ, Martinez FJ, Anzueto A, Barnes PJ, Bourbeau J, et al. Global strategy for the diagnosis, management, and prevention of chronic obstructive lung disease 2017 report: GOLD executive summary. Archivos de Bronconeumología. 2017;**53**(3):128-149. Epub 2017/03/10. DOI: 10.1016/j.arbres.2017.02.001

[58] Crim C, Dransfield MT, Bourbeau J, Jones PW, Hanania NA, Mahler DA, et al. Pneumonia risk with inhaled fluticasone furoate and vilanterol compared with vilanterol alone in patients with COPD. Annals of the American Thoracic Society. 2015;**12**(1):27-34. Epub 2014/12/10. DOI: 10.1513/AnnalsATS.201409-413OC

[59] Singh S, Loke YK. Risk of pneumonia associated with long-term use of inhaled corticosteroids in chronic obstructive pulmonary disease: A critical review and update. Current Opinion in Pulmonary Medicine. 2010;**16**(2):118-122. Epub 2009/11/21. DOI: 10.1097/MCP.0b013e328334c085

[60] Yang IA, Fong KM, Sim EH, Black PN, Lasserson TJ. Inhaled corticosteroids for stable chronic obstructive pulmonary disease. Cochrane Database of Systematic Reviews. 2007;**(2)**:Cd002991. Epub 2007/04/20. DOI: 10.1002/14651858.CD002991.pub2

[61] Shafiek H, Verdú J, Iglesias A, Ramon-Clar L, Toledo-Pons N, Lopez-Causape C, et al. Inhaled corticosteroid dose is associated with Pseudomonas aeruginosa infection in severe COPD. BMJ Open Respir Res. 2021;**8**(1). Epub 2021/10/08. DOI: 10.1136/bmjresp-2021-001067

[62] Cerón-Pisa N, Shafiek H, Martín-Medina A, Verdú J, Jordana-Lluch E, Escobar-Salom M, et al. Effects of Inhaled Corticosteroids on the Innate Immunological Response to Pseudomonas aeruginosa Infection in Patients with COPD. Int J Mol Sci. 2022;**23**(15). Epub 2022/07/29. DOI: 10.3390/ijms23158127

[63] O'Byrne PM, Pedersen S, Carlsson LG, Radner F, Thorén A, Peterson S, et al. Risks of pneumonia in patients with asthma taking inhaled corticosteroids. American Journal of Respiratory and Critical Care Medicine. 2011;**183**(5):589-595. Epub 2010/10/05. DOI: 10.1164/rccm.201005-0694OC

[64] Qian CJ, Coulombe J, Suissa S, Ernst P. Pneumonia risk in asthma patients using inhaled corticosteroids: A quasi-cohort study. British Journal of Clinical Pharmacology. 2017;**83**(9):2077-2086. Epub 2017/04/21. DOI: 10.1111/bcp.13295

[65] You Y, Ni Y, Shi G. Inhaled corticosteroids and mycobacterial infection in patients with chronic airway diseases: A systematic review and meta-analysis. Respiration. 2022;**101**(10):970-980. Epub 2022/08/24. DOI: 10.1159/000525980

[66] Loke YK, Cavallazzi R, Singh S. Risk of fractures with inhaled corticosteroids in COPD: Systematic review and meta-analysis of randomised controlled trials and observational studies. Thorax. 2011;**66**(8):699-708. Epub 2011/05/24. DOI: 10.1136/thx.2011.160028

[67] Lehouck A, Boonen S, Decramer M, Janssens W. COPD, bone metabolism, and osteoporosis. Chest. 2011;**139**(3):648-657. Epub 2011/03/03. DOI: 10.1378/chest.10-1427

[68] Barnes PJ, Pedersen S, Busse WW. Efficacy and safety of inhaled corticosteroids. New developments. American Journal of Respiratory and Critical Care Medicine. 1998;**157**(3 Pt 2):S1-S53. Epub 1998/04/01. DOI: 10.1164/ajrccm.157.3.157315

[69] Suissa S, Kezouh A, Ernst P. Inhaled corticosteroids and the risks of diabetes onset and progression. The American Journal of Medicine. 2010;**123**(11):1001-1006. Epub 2010/09/28. DOI: 10.1016/j.amjmed.2010.06.019

[70] Wang JJ, Rochtchina E, Tan AG, Cumming RG, Leeder SR, Mitchell P. Use of inhaled and oral corticosteroids and the long-term risk of cataract. Ophthalmology. 2009;**116**(4):652-657. Epub 2009/02/27. DOI: 10.1016/j.ophtha.2008.12.001

[71] Garbe E, LeLorier J, Boivin JF, Suissa S. Inhaled and nasal glucocorticoids and the risks of ocular hypertension or open-angle glaucoma. Journal of the American Medical Association. 1997;**277**(9):722-727 Epub 1997/03/05

Chapter 4

Drug Delivery of Corticosteroids

Mohamed S. El-Khooly

Abstract

In this chapter, we will study how we were able to place drugs from the family of corticosteroids in the places where the drug is intended to be affected during the surgery. It was also possible to control the release of accumulated quantities of dexamethasone by coating it with some soluble polymers such as chitosan. We used samples of bioglass grafted with chitosan polymer to which different percentages of dexamethasone (Dexa) were added (5, 10, and 15%). In addition, the cumulative doses emitted from the samples were calculated by means of statistical functions and using the ultraviolet device. This was also tested on the plasma fluid of the human-simulating body fluid (SBF), and it was confirmed that the appropriate amounts of Dexa were emitted over a period of (1, 2, 4, 8, 16, 21, and 33) days. Due to its shown efficacy in simulating in liquid of the human body (SBF), we aim to put it within the human body as soon as feasible.

Keywords: DDS, stander curve, dexamethasone release, SBF, chitosan

1. Introduction

Corticosteroid drug delivery is a brand-new, fast-developing area in medical research. A corticosteroid-like dexamethasone is a suitable bioactive compound that may be used in bone tissue engineering applications. However, using drug delivery technology today is known to be crucial because it prevents the medications from passing through GIT. Additionally, this medication may be used in an osteogenic medium to encourage the development of stem cells that follow the osteogenic lineage [1–3].

Biodegradable polymers are thought to be the best choice for biological applications in tissue engineering and drug delivery, where the characteristics of bioactive glass can be enhanced and drug release patterns can be changed when polymers are utilized in bioactive glass/polymer composites. Accordingly, to increase patient compliance, the capacity of long-term medication administration for treating chronic illnesses would be crucial. By utilizing bioactive glass/polymer composites, various medications may be locally released and drug delivery systems already have employed a variety of medications, including anti-inflammatory, osteogenic, anticancer, and antibiotics [4, 5]. The characteristics of bioactive glass can be enhanced and drug release patterns can be changed when polymers are utilized in bioactive glass/polymer composites [6]. Due to the widespread usage of dexamethasone as anti-inflammatory medicine, we attempted to create a novel drug delivery system based on (chitosan and bioglass) [7].

This study aims to create and describe solid lipid nanoparticles (SLNs) loaded with Dexa-P and compare them to other drugs with a similar structure or lipophilicity demonstrating that utilizing Dexa-P increases medication loading in SLNs. The development of the standard operating procedure for preparation allowed for evaluation of the size, form, structure, and crystallinity of SLNs.

2. Drug delivery systems (DDS)

2.1 Definition

Technologies that release medications and bioactive chemicals are referred to regarded as "drug delivery" in general (e.g., proteins, growth factors, lipids, genes) [8] . Typically, it involves a substance that delivers the medication to the targeted area and keeps the therapeutic agent there. This substance is frequently referred to as the system's carrier or matrix. The idea of controlled release has, more often than not, been closely linked to the idea of medication delivery. A medicinal drug is delivered and released in a time-dependent way under the term "controlled release." This continuous release is necessary since it influences the dosage that a patient should take and how quickly an organism absorbs the medication [9, 10].

2.2 Therapeutic window

The boundaries between the minimum toxic concentration (MTC) and the lowest effective concentration are known as the therapeutic window (MEC). MTC serves as an upper limit since it is the lowest concentration necessary to cause a living thing to exhibit hazardous behavior. MEC, on the other hand, functions as a lower limit since the intended effect is produced at the minimal concentration. Therefore, to sustain the medicine's efficacy without causing a hazardous reaction, the drug concentration must constantly remain within the therapeutic window [11].

2.3 Historical perspective

The first implant, released in 1989, disperses goserelin acetate over a one- to three-month period. Less than 10 clinical treatments that deliver additional peptides and proteins have since been developed, highlighting the challenges in product development. The second generation's final 10 years were devoted to the creation of medication delivery devices based on nanotechnology. The technologies indicated in **Table 1** represent the second generation of drug delivery, which has not yet been created. However, in order for the third generation of medication delivery to be successful, it must address and get over the problems that the first two generations of drug delivery systems have. The three generations of medication delivery are listed in **Table 1**. Smith Kline & French developed the first controlled release medication in 1952 for dextroamphetamine distribution over a 12-hour period (Dexedrine) [12].

2.4 Future back

It is impossible to forecast the developments in medication delivery technology that will occur over the next 30 years. No matter what new technologies are created, our existing demands for treating illnesses and overcoming obstacles to better

Year: 1950–1980	1980–2010	2010–2040
1st Generation	**2nd Generation**	**3rd Generation**
Basics of controlled release	Smart delivery systems	Modulated delivery systems
Oral delivery Twice-a-day or once-a-day	Zero-order release Zero vs first-order release	On-off insulin release Glucose-sensitive release
Transdermal delivery Once-a-day, once-a-week	Smart polymers & hydrogels Environment-sensitive Self-regulated release	Targeted delivery Anticancer drugs, siRNA
Drug release mechanisms Dissolution, diffusion, osmosis, and ion-exchange	Peptide & protein delivery Biodegradable depot	Long-term delivery systems 6–12 months with the minimal initial burst effect
	Nanoparticles Tumor-targeted delivery Gene delivery	In vitro-In vivo correlation Prediction of PK profiles from in vitro release study

Table 1.
Evolution of controlled drug delivery systems.

medicine delivery will remain the same. The issues described will need to be resolved by more advanced medication delivery technology (**Table 1**).

As the number of people with diabetes keeps growing, there will be a greater need for designing modified insulin delivery devices. Since more than 10 years ago, targeted medicine delivery to tumors has been a major area of study. This demand will not go away overnight. To increase patient compliance, the capacity of long-term medication administration, that is, 6 months or longer, for treating chronic illnesses, would be crucial. Additionally, novel *in vitro* testing techniques will need to be created to precisely forecast the human *in vivo* pharmacokinetics of medicines and drug formulations. Scientists working on drug delivery can wait and see what new technologies are created in the future to address the current issues. But with this passive attitude, we will not be able to meet our objectives in a timely manner. Instead, medicine delivery researchers might use a daring new strategy called "future back." The future back method focuses on comprehending what is plainly achievable or impossible rather than trying to imagine the future to discover a means to accomplish a goal. Scientists will only be able to advance to the level of the norms and priorities of that period if they rely on future inventions that have not yet been created. This is particularly true when innovations are in small scale and soon become obsolete [13].

To reach the aim, scientists may specify what innovations are required and how to combine those breakthroughs to create the perfect drug delivery system. This allows them to start by describing an ideal drug delivery system with all desirable qualities.

At least four modified delivery mechanisms will be developed during the third generation. The targeted delivery of anticancer drugs or siRNA to tumors, the glucose-sensitive transient insulin delivery with on-off switching capability, the long-term drug delivery ranging from 6 months to 1 year, and *in vitro* testing techniques that can predict *in vivo* pharmacokinetic profiles are among them. Technically speaking, creating a modified insulin delivery system, is the most difficult of them.

Delivering insulin is distinct from administering other medications in that it must be administered at the appropriate moment, that is, when the blood glucose level rises, and in a precise quantity that is just sufficient to lower the blood glucose level.

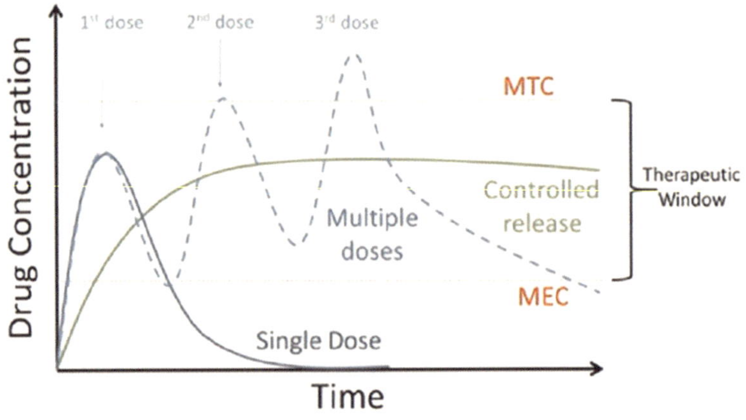

Figure 1.
Therapeutic window are the limits between the minimum toxic concentration (MTC) and the minimum effective concentration (MEC). Single-dose drug concentration in the plasma (blue solid line), multiple-dose drug concentration in the plasma (dotted line), and zero-order controlled release (green solid line) in the therapeutic window. The range in which a pharmacological dose is effective without having a toxic impact is defined as the area between the minimum toxic concentration (MTC) and the minimum effective concentration (MEC).

The insulin level in the blood should pulse rather than remain constant, as seen in **Figure 1**. Following a drop in glucose levels, the blood's insulin concentration should also drop.

Hypoglycemia will happen otherwise. Pulsatile drug release systems that are practical for clinical applications still need to be developed despite substantial advancements [14].

2.5 DDS advantages and disadvantages

2.5.1 Advantages

Increasing the drug's bioavailability and duration of effect.

Little medication loss and degradation.

Preventing harmful medicine side effects.

Lowering the dosage frequency.

Medication consumption is improved and drug concentration variations are minimized in plasma levels.

Patient compliance has improved.

2.5.2 Disadvantages

Products of harmful degradation.

Patients' pain with the use of the DDS device necessitates surgical Intervention, either for the installation or removal of systems.

High price of the finished item.

2.6 Mechanisms of drug release

There are a number of ways that a substance might release a drug; here, we will concentrate on the most common ones. The two primary categories of these mechanisms are non-responsive and responsive. Non-responsive systems, in which the therapeutic agent is released as a result of matrix swelling or disintegration, do not require an external stimulus to deliver a medicine. The following is a list of ineffective methods [15].

2.6.1 Diffusion mechanism

It is based on how water (from bodily fluid) and the matrix where the medicine is loaded interact. Monolithic and reservoir matrices are the two types of matrices that adhere to this principle. This carrier is referred to be a monolithic matrix if the medicine is evenly distributed throughout the matrix and is able to diffuse *via* the pores when the matrix breaks down. If not, the matrix is categorized as a reservoir because the medication is disseminated through a coating layer that covers its surface. The superficial layer in reservoir matrices therefore regulates the release kinetics. Typically, both systems exhibit a burst release followed by zero-order kinetics.

2.6.2 Controlled osmosis

Osmotic pressure acts as the driving force to disperse the drug outward from the matrix when the difference in drug concentration is between the matrix and the surrounding fluid. The kinetics of this process frequently has zero order.

2.6.3 Ionic exchange

It is connected to ionic medications that replenish ions in live tissue *via* a concentration gradient or it is associated with ionic drugs that restore the ions in living tissue along a gradient of concentration.

2.6.4 Erosion mechanism

It is dependent on the matrix's degradation. It is divided into two stages:

Therapeutic compounds can then be released under zero-order kinetics after the matrix has first undergone a superficial degradation. As the matrix dissolves over time and the bulk degrades with time, drug release is also facilitated. Sensitive medications may often be supplied primarily in the target tissue and avoid their early degradation if the first stage is under control.

2.7 Materials in drug delivery systems

2.7.1 Ceramics for biomedical applications

Bioceramics have long been used as bone grafting for applications involving bone regeneration. Only the bioactive ceramics (such as hydroxyapatite, bioactive glass, and glass ceramics) and the resorbable ceramics (such as tricalcium phosphate and biocompatible glasses) are suitable for bone regeneration applications as scaffolds because they permit the adherence and proliferation of cells from the host tissue. This is true even though the class of ceramic biomaterials includes bioinert, bioactive, and resorbable ceramics [16].

2.7.2 Polymers in drug delivery systems

As previously indicated, DDS can be made utilizing synthetic or natural polymers that are either biodegradable or not (see **Figure 2**). Drugs, proteins, and cells can all be released using these polymeric systems. As mentioned in the preceding section, the polymers employed in DDS should exhibit a variety of characteristics that make them ideal materials to interact with the human body, with biodegradability being one of the most crucial characteristics.

Both swelling and osmosis can be used to manage solvent-activated systems. A hydrophilic polymeric crosslinked chain that can absorb a lot of water without dissolving is the foundation of systems that control swelling. The quantity of water that enters the polymeric matrix determines how quickly the medicine inside the system diffuses outward thanks to this water absorption (shown in **Figure 3**). Systems that are controlled by osmosis rely on a device.

Numerous dissolved or degradable polymers are appropriate for use in medication delivery systems. The timing of the medication release or release outside the prepared material is managed in terms of the rate of water absorption and disintegration. The polymer's high molecular weight and viscosity are blamed for the departure. Chitosan,

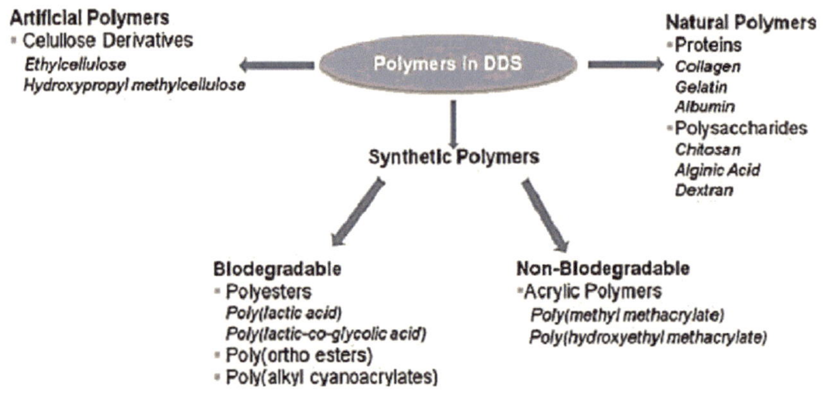

Figure 2.
Overview of the polymers used in drug delivery systems [44].

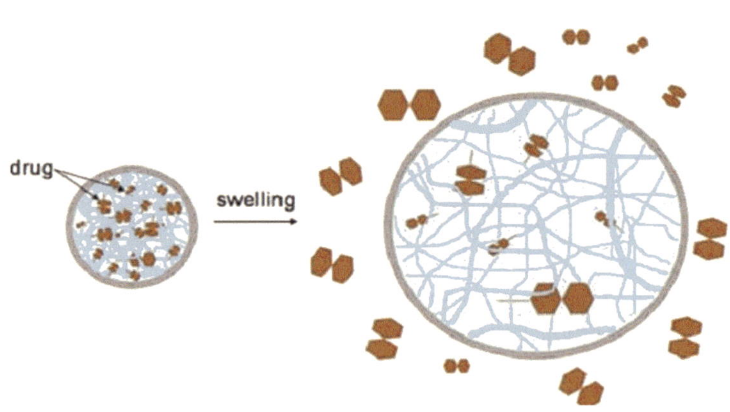

Figure 3.
Drug release resulting from swelling of a polymeric matrix containing a DDS, without or with small amount of drug flows toward a chamber in which the drug is contained [17].

sodium alginate, and zein protein are the three most well-known polymers utilized in this field.

2.7.3 Polysaccharides

Monosaccharide-repeating units are the building blocks of polysaccharides, which are high-molecular-weight compounds. They provide a wide variety of structures and attributes. The variety of possible uses is increased by reactive lateral groups, which allows for the changing of their structure. Dextran, alginate, and chitosan are a few of the materials that are typically used to make DDS.

A polysaccharide of bacterial origin, dextran is mostly made up of 1,6-linked D-glucopyranose units. It could have side branches at the positions α-1,2-, α-1,3-, or α-1,4 (**Figure 4**) [18].

2.7.3.1 Chitosan

Chitosan, a cationic polymer created by the alkaline deacetylation of chitin, is the primary component of marine crab shells (see **Figure 5**). According to a review by Thu Ta and co-authors, chitosan-based hydrogels have been employed as DDS in the field of cancer therapy. There were many preparation techniques and crosslinking agents presented. Paclitaxel, doxorubicin, and camptothecin are a few examples of entrapped medicines [19].

2.8 Bioactive glass/polymer composites

Different material classes each have advantages and drawbacks of their own. For instance, bioactive glasses and other ceramic materials exhibit good biocompatibility, compression resistance, and corrosion resistance, but they have issues such as brittleness, low fracture strength, and high density. Polymers, on the other hand, may have a variety of forms, compositions, and physical characteristics, but they are too flexible and weak for some applications [20].

In this way, composite materials comprised of ceramic and polymers combine the benefits of each type of material while also addressing their drawbacks. In addition to

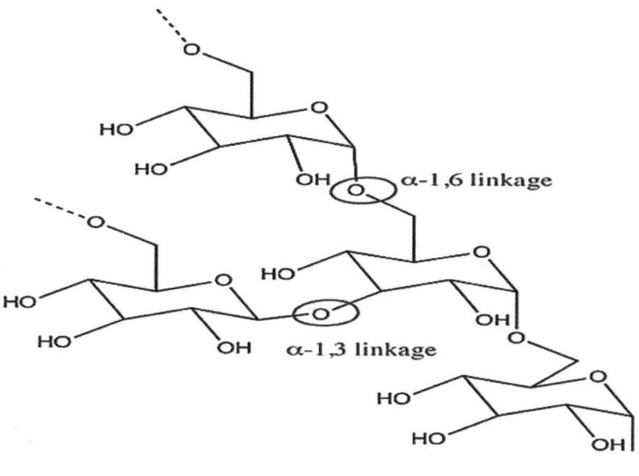

Figure 4.
Molecular structure of dextran.

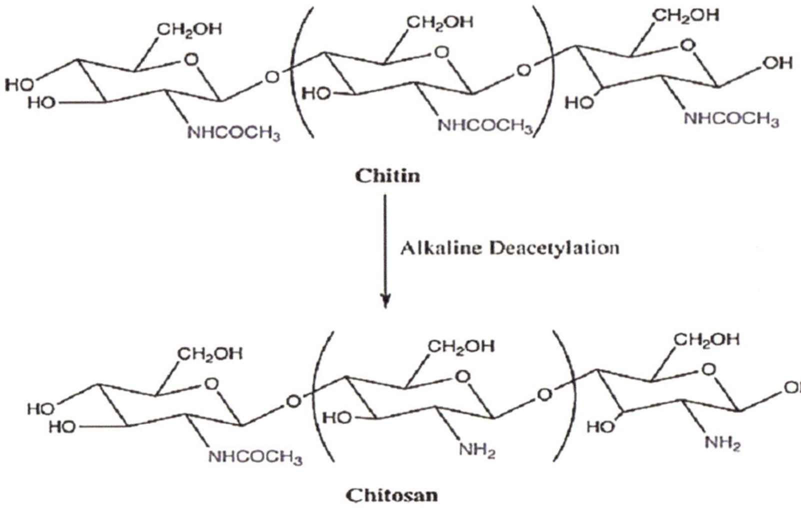

Figure 5.
Schematic representation of the alkaline deacetylation of chitin to obtain chitosan.

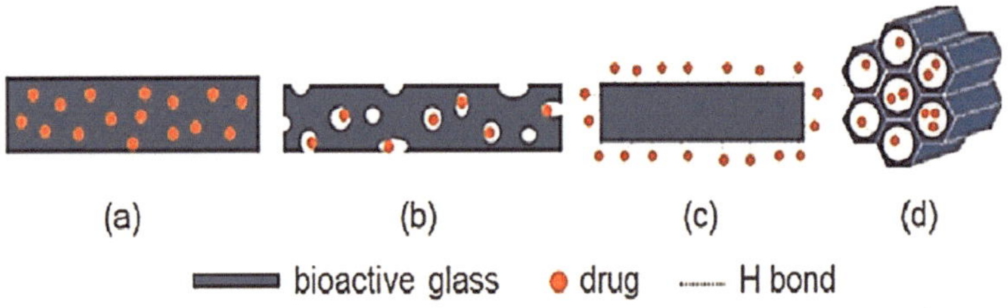

Figure 6.
Schematic diagrams of: (a) drug incorporated during sol-gel syntheses of BG; (b) drug entrapped inside porous of bioactive glass; (c) drug bonded by H bond on surface of BG; and (d) drug bonded by H bond on inner surface of mesoporous BG.

modifying drug release patterns, polymers utilized in bioactive glass/polymer composites can enhance the mechanical and physical characteristics of bioactive glasses [6]. On the other hand, bioactive glass particles incorporated into polymers boost the material's bioactivity while also improving mechanical performance [4]. The medication can be put in either the glass or the polymeric matrix in these devices. Drug loading in polymers is accomplished by incorporating medicines into a polymer matrix [21].

There are two ways that the medicine can be put into the glass particles (**Figure 6**): bioactive glass (BG) and bioactive glass with mesopores (MBG) [22].

Different morphologies, such as the dispersion of bioactive glass particles into a polymeric matrix or polymeric fibers, the coating of a polymer on the surface of a bioactive glass scaffold, or the coating of bioactive glass particles on the surface of a polymeric scaffold, can result in the association of polymers with bioactive glass. Each system has distinct mechanical traits and capabilities and may be used for specialized tasks (**Figure 7**).

2.9 Clinical applications of bioactive glass/polymer for DDS

Utilizing bioactive glass/polymer composites, various medications may be locally released. Drug delivery systems have employed a variety of medications, including

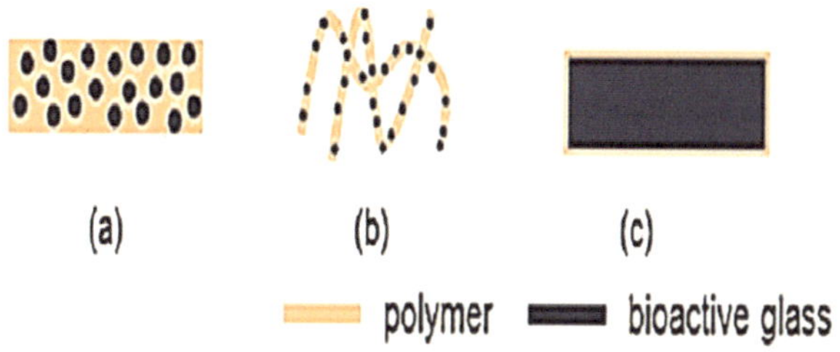

Figure 7.
Schematic diagrams of: (a) bioactive glass particles in a polymeric matrix; (b) bioactive glass particles in polymeric fibers; (c) coating of a bioactive glass scaffold with polymer; and (d) coating of a polymeric scaffold with bioactive glasses particles.

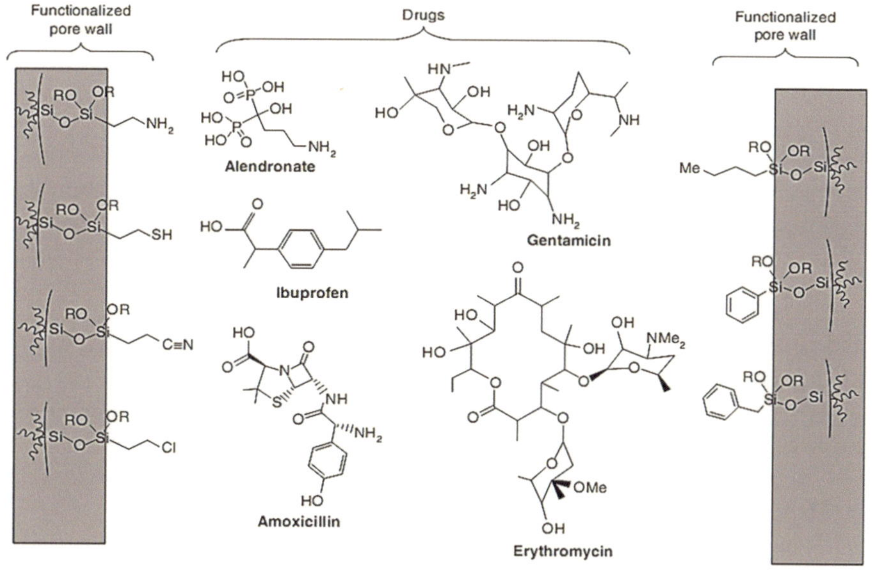

Figure 8.
Exemplifies functionalized pore wall of mesoporous.

anti-inflammatory, osteogenic, anticancer, and antibiotics. This section will discuss various uses for these medications put into glass or polymer matrixes (seen in **Figure 8**) [23].

2.10 Antibiotics in DDS

Since the use of biomaterials like bone fillers, bone substitutes, or orthopedic implants may have unfavorable outcomes like infections, antibiotics make up the majority of the medications used in local release. Because the osteogenic response of glass and the drug release by the composite may be combined, employing glass/polymer scaffolds is preferable to using glass and polymers separately. Additionally, substantial medication dosages can be locally released, improving the treatment's specificity. This capacity is necessary for bone infections like osteomyelitis because it enables the diffusion of high dosages of antibiotics to avascular regions that the systemic administration cannot [24]. Numerous studies have suggested various bioactive glass/polymer scaffolds for releasing antibiotics.

2.11 Anti-inflammatory in DDS

Inflammatory reactions are frequently seen following surgery or implant procedures. Anti-inflammatory medicine local release may be a solution to reduce this issue.

Anti-inflammatory responses are crucial for tissue regeneration because they aid in the removal of foreign infections, but if they are too strong, they can harm the tissue.

2.12 DDS used to cancer treatment

Bone cancer is another issue that causes a reduction in bone mass. Chemotherapy, which involves administering one or more medications systemically to cancer cells, is a common treatment for bone cancer. Chemotherapy has a drawback: Side effects can harm patients' quality of life and have an overall unfavorable impact on their bodies. For the treatment of bone cancer, local medication administration may enhance the medicine's activity against cancer cells and minimize or eliminate adverse effects. The interaction with bioactive eyewear may potentially promote the repair of damaged tissue (**Figure 9**).

Recombinant granulocyte colony-stimulating factor treatment showed a diminished impact, while recombinant granulocyte-macrophage colony-stimulating factor had no encouraging impact. Recombinant granulocyte-macrophage colony-stimulating factor, on the other hand, increased acute myeloid leukemia incidence (by 75%), while colony-stimulating factor 1 and recombinant granulocyte colony stimulating factor had no effect. This was discovered when different factors were administered several months after the leukemogenic treatment. Recombinant interleukin 6 treatment, on the other hand, significantly (23%) decreased the risk of acute myeloid leukemia. The results show that radiation-induced preleukemia, a component of radiation-induced acute myeloid leukemia in mice, is a multiphase process [25].

2.13 Multifunctional drug delivery systems

In addition to coatings, in more sophisticated systems, such medication delivery systems have also been created: synthetic macro- and mesoporous silica Santa Barbara Amorphous (SBA-15) with magnetic particle-filled porous bioactive glass (magnetic

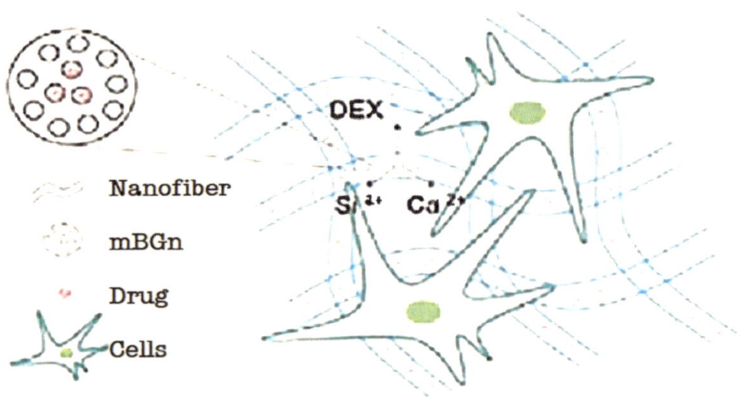

Figure 9.
Schematic diagram showing the therapeutic fiber scaffolds incorporating nanospheres of mesoporous bioactive glass with dexamethasone (Dexa-loaded mBGn), where the drug releasing effect and bioactivity of mBGn can be synergized to regulate osteogenic responses.

SBA-15). After being submerged in a hexane/ibuprofen solution to load the anti-inflammatory medication ibuprofen, magnetic SBA-15 was coated with polymer (lactic-co-glycolic acid). The diabetic medication metformin HCl was then added to bioactive glasses. *In vitro* testing revealed the release characteristics of both medications [26].

2.14 Why glucocorticoids in DDS

Drugs called glucocorticoids, sometimes known as corticosteroids or "steroids," are particularly efficient in reducing inflammation brought on by ailments such as asthma and arthritis. They may also be administered to replace the body's own natural steroids in cases of pituitary or adrenal illness. Prednisolone and dexamethasone are the two glucocorticoids that are most often utilized. They typically play a crucial role in the management of numerous medical problems and have the potential to save lives. However, doctors often utilize the lowest amount necessary to manage the disease and only suggest them when it is truly essential.

2.15 How do they affect bone?

One of the known adverse effects of glucocorticoid therapy is that it might weaken bones and increase the likelihood of fractures, especially when used for an extended length of time. Both direct and indirect actions of glucocorticoids on bone contribute to bone loss and decreased bone strength.

By promoting the activity of natural bone removal cells and decreasing the activity of bone-building cells, they have a detrimental effect on bone directly. They may also impact the amounts of sex hormones and the way the body processes calcium. The degree of bone loss varies from person to person, but for individuals taking 7.5 mg or more of prednisolone per day, the risk of fractures rises by more than 50% in the first year of treatment.

2.16 Do all glucocorticoid treatments affect bone?

The dosage of glucocorticoids and how they are administered both affect how they affect bones throughout treatment (as an injection, cream, inhaler). But glucocorticoid medications are the ones that have been most closely linked to bone loss. Although studies indicate that increased fracture risk can occur even with modest doses of prednisolone (2.5–7.5 mg per day) and climb further with increasing daily dosages, the precise quantity that is damaging to bone varies depending on the individual. Another important factor is how long glucocorticoid pills are taken. The majority of specialists concur that there may be an effect on bone if they are used constantly in tablet form for longer than 3 months. If extremely large dosages are utilized, this impact can be seen much sooner. The overall health advantages of glucocorticoids far outweigh any potential slight negative effect on bones when they are used in low doses to replace what the body is unable to produce (e.g., in Addison's disease or pituitary disease), so it is crucial that they are taken as prescribed by your doctor [27].

2.17 Dexamethasone (Dexa)

Additional medications may be given either before or simultaneously with the chemotherapeutic medicines to lessen or eliminate these chemotherapy resistance

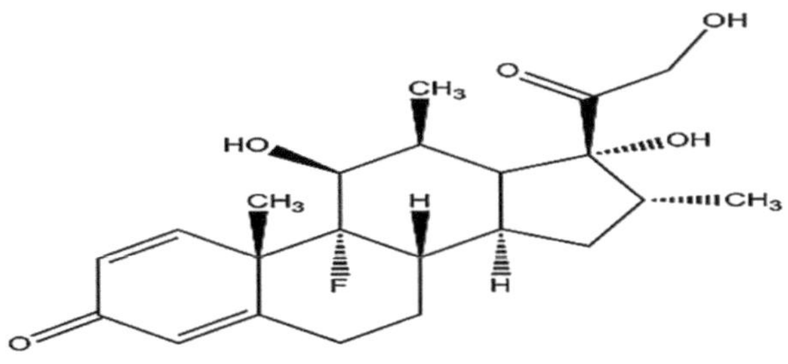

Figure 10.
Structures of dexamethasone.

factors. These medications may or may not have therapeutic benefits on their own, but their main function is as adjuvants, enhancing the effectiveness and/or reducing the toxicity of chemotherapeutic medicines. Dexa (**Figure 10**) is one such medication. Synthetic glucocorticoids like Dexa are well known for their ability to reduce inflammation and suppress the immune system. It has demonstrated benefit against several malignancies, including leukemia, and has been widely used as an anti-emetic in combination with chemotherapy drugs [28].

However, recent preclinical and clinical studies have concentrated on its use as a chemotherapeutic adjuvant. According to studies, pretreatment with Dexa can lessen the toxicity and, in some situations, boost the effectiveness of chemotherapy drugs. Prednisolone and Dexa, for instance, both efficiently defended progenitor cells in four strains of mice against 5-fluorouracil, a chemotherapeutic drug that is specific to the cell cycle and is antimetabolic. Blood cell counts and the number of bone marrow progenitors both returned to normal after 3–5 days and 1–2 days, respectively, of not receiving glucocorticoids. With Dexa, the same degree of effectiveness may be attained at almost 16.5 times the dosage of prednisolone.

In six xenograft models studied (2 colon, 2 breast, 1 lung, and 1 glioma tumors), Wang et al. found that pre-administration of Dexa was able to greatly boost the effectiveness of carboplatin, a DNA alkylating agent; gemcitabine, an antimetabolite; or a combination of both medicines by 2–4-fold. The same team also looked at how Dexa affected the treatment with Adriamycin, an anthracycline antibiotic that may intercalate DNA and is also known as doxorubicin, with similar outcomes. In a syngeneic model of breast cancer, pre-administration of Dexa led to an almost total suppression of tumor development. Dexa pretreatment has been shown in clinical studies to decrease hematological toxicity and speed up the recovery of absolute granulocyte count and platelet count [29].

By employing normal phase LC with quaternary mobile phase with regulated water content, UV detection at 254 nm, and cortisone as an internal standard, dexamethasone content in drug substance and elixir may be found. In bulk drug material and elixir, TLC, IR spectroscopy, and relative LC retention time ratios are used to validate identification.

2.18 Dexamethasone interactions

Dexamethasone's role in treating rats with gastrointestinal constipation brought on by morphine, verapamil, and atropine has been investigated. Dexamethasone was able to counteract the dose-related inhibition of charcoal meal transit brought on by these medications. More effectively than altering the effects of verapamil, dexamethasone reversed the constipation caused by morphine and atropine. Dexamethasone's interaction with its receptor was shown to have the potential to release a greater amount of acetylcholine, which would reverse the constipation caused by atropine or morphine. Dexamethasone's little impact on verapamil-induced constipation revealed that calcium influx was not as important as previously thought. The aforementioned findings point to the significance of steroids in gastrointestinal transit and offer a potential mechanism by which dexamethasone might alleviate constipation brought on by morphine and atropine [30].

2.19 Dexamethasone health hazard

SYMPTOMS Fluid and electrolyte disturbances, pituitary-adrenal suppression, hyperglycemia, increased susceptibility to infection, including tuberculosis, myopathy, growth arrest, hypokalemic alkalosis, and Cushing's syndrome, which includes "moon-face," "buffalo-hump," striae, acne, and hirsutism, are all symptoms of exposure to this type of compound. Ecchymoses, "central obesity," and enlarged supraclavicular fat pads are some additional signs of Cushing's syndrome.

This condition can also lead to increased bruising and flushing. Behavioral abnormalities, glycosuria, anxiousness, mood or psyche changes, psychopathy's of the manic-depressive or schizophrenia type, and suicidal thoughts are further signs of exposure. Candidiasis, gluconeogenesis, heart failure (in severe cases), spontaneous fractures, increased hunger, slower wound healing, hyperhidrosis, neurological and mental problems, intracranial hypertension, and increased blood coagulability are all possible side effects of exposure. Aseptic necrosis of the bone, amenorrhea, muscle weakness, salt and water retention, hypertension, edema, increased severity of diabetes, pancreatitis, thrombotic episodes, and osteoporosis are other possible side effects. Sleeplessness, skin eruptions, depression, euphoria, decreased pain perception, weakness, deafness, convulsions, intestinal perforation in ulcerative colitis, hypokalemia, muscle deterioration, Achilles tendon rupture, pseudotumor cerebri, and cardiac conduction defect are additional signs of exposure to this type of substance.

Congestive heart failure, immune system suppression, impaired glucose tolerance, habituation, and the emergence of hidden psychological disorders are among its potential side effects. Additionally, it may result in potassium loss, muscle mass loss, vertebral compression fractures, abdominal distention, ulcerative esophagitis, thin and fragile skin, petechiae, erythema, increased sweating, suppressed skin test reactions, allergic dermatitis, urticaria, angioneurotic edema, vertigo, headache, decreased carbohydrate tolerance, exophthalmos, hypersensitivity, thromboembolism, malnutrition. Ascites may occur. Subcutaneous atrophy and skin collagen loss might result from skin exposure to this kind of substance. Burning, secondary infections, itching, irritation, pigmentation, dryness, folliculitis, and hypertrichosis are additional signs of this approach. This kind of chemical can cause cataracts, increased intraocular pressure, corneal ulcers, and impaired vision in the eyes. Glaucoma might also happen [31].

2.20 Acute/chronic hazards

Through consumption, inhalation, or skin absorption, this substance may be dangerous. It could irritate others. It could result in lacrimation. It releases deadly fumes of carbon monoxide, carbon dioxide, and hydrogen fluoride when heated to the point of disintegration [32, 33].

2.21 Dexamethasone chemical dangers

When heated over 275°C, it decomposes. This releases harmful gases. This creates a risk of fire and explosion, and reacts with carbon disulfide, copper, lead, silver, mercury, and other metals. Particularly shock-sensitive chemicals are created as a result and with acids reacts. As a result, poisonous and explosive hydrogen aside is produced, with a melting point between 504 and 507 degrees F. [25, 34].

2.22 Preparation of drug-loaded SLNs

It has been demonstrated that using Dexa-P improves medication loading in solid lipid nanoparticles (SLNs). This section's objectives were to manufacture and describe SLNs that were loaded with Dexa-P and to compare them to other medications with a comparable structure or lipophilicity. Size, form, structure, and crystallinity of SLNs will be evaluated, in addition to the previously mentioned characteristics (drug loading and encapsulation effectiveness). The free and encapsulated medication will be separated using ultrafiltration, and the amount will be measured using an HPLC-UV test. For the comparative experiments, curcumin and ascorbic palmitate (AP) will be employed. The palmitate moiety that may link with the SLN lipids is absent from curcumin, despite the fact that both medicines are lipophilic.

2.23 Stability of drug-loaded SLNs

The presence of CE activity seems to be necessary for the release of dexa from the SLNs. This section's objectives were to 1) establish the stability of SLNs and 2) demonstrate dexa-P retention with the SLNs in circumstances similar to those in human plasma (specifically the absence of CE activity). Monitoring the growth and morphology of SLNs cultured at 37°C was the main goal of the early experiments. The influence of SLN concentration on particle size growth was assessed, and SLNs returned to 4°C after incubation at 37°C were tested for size recovery to better clarify the process of particle size growth. After that, SLNs were exposed to human serum albumin (HSA), and a representative protein, and size and turbidity alterations were observed. As a backup strategy, size exclusion chromatography (SEC) was applied to validate the SLNs' intact status in the presence of HSA. A multi-step filtration procedure that involved first filtering *via* a 0.2-μm membrane and then ultrafiltration was used to ascertain the retention of Dexa-P with the SLNs in the presence of human plasma. Calculating the quantity of medication retained with the SLNs involved taking into consideration the known protein binding.

2.24 Storage stability of drug-loaded SLNs

This section's objectives were to examine the long-term stability of aqueous and lyophilized SLNs and to optimize a process for lyophilizing SLNs. The following factors were taken into account for optimizing the lyophilization protocol: lyoprotectant (LP) type and concentration, SLN concentration, freezing temperature, freezing rate, and drying time. The particle size, shape, mono dispersity, and drug loading of SLNs were evaluated. Lyophilized SLNs and SLN suspensions were kept at 4°C and 25°C/60% RH for the long-term stability testing. At days 0, 1, 3, 7, 14, and months 1, 2, and 3, samples were taken to evaluate the size of the particles and drug loading [35].

2.25 Biological activity

It is permitted to use dexamethasone to lessen immunological response and minimize inflammation. The following cancers are treated with it in combination with other medications: leukemia, lymphoma, fungus mycoides (a type of cutaneous T-cell lymphoma). The following cancer-related diseases are also prevented or treated using dexamethasone alone or in combination with other medications: anemia, cerebral edema (fluid build-up in the brain) (fluid build-up in the brain), hypersensitivity to drugs (allergic reactions), hypercalcemia (high blood levels of calcium) (high blood levels of calcium), thrombocytopenia (low platelet levels) (low platelet levels). Many different illnesses and ailments are treated with dexamethasone either on its own or in combination with other medications. The medication is still being researched for the treatment of many cancers and other illnesses [36].

2.26 Therapeutic uses

Dexamethasone is mostly utilized as an immunosuppressant or anti-inflammatory drug. The medication is insufficient by itself to treat adrenocortical insufficiency because it only possesses limited mineralocorticoid characteristics. Dexamethasone must be administered in conjunction with a mineralocorticoid to effectively treat this disease: steroidal anti-inflammatory drugs, antiemetics, hormonal antineoplastics, synthetic and topical glucocorticoids, and antihistamine [37].

In babies and children with Haemophiles influenzae meningitis, there is some evidence that short-term supplementary treatment with IV dexamethasone may reduce the incidence of audiologic and/or neurologic sequelae. Patients with *Streptococcus pneumoniae* meningitis may also benefit. The American Academy of Pediatrics (AAP) and other medical professionals advise considering adjunctive dexamethasone therapy in infants and kids older than 6 weeks with known or suspected bacterial meningitis, particularly in those with suspected or confirmed *Haemophilus influenzae* infection, during the first 2–4 days of anti-infective therapy. Dexamethasone should be started before or concurrently with the initial dosage of an anti-infective medication if it is used [38].

3. *In vitro* bioactive analysis

3.1 Standard operating procedure for (SBF) preparation

Kokubo's [39] Simulated body fluid (SBF) is a metastable solution made up of supersaturated calcium and phosphate ions in relation to apatite.

As a result, (SBF) is ready as follows:

- The buffer solution with pH values between 4 and 7 was used to calibrate the pH meter.
- The procedure is conducted with the temperature at 37.4°C.
- SBF solution was created by combining the listed components in the right amounts and sequence (as specified in **Table 2**) in 950 ml of distilled water.

Order	Reagent	Amount (g/L)	Formula weight
1	Tris	6.057	121.1356
2	HCl	39 (ml)	—
3	NaCl	8.006	58.44277
4	$NaHCO_3$	0.352	84.00687
5	KCl	0.223	74.551
6	$K_2HPO_4.3H_2O$	0.228	228.222
7	$CaCl_2$	0.277	110.986
8	Na_2SO_4	0.071	142.03714
9	$MgCl_2.6H_2O$	0.304	203.3034

Table 2.
Reagents for preparation of simulated body fluid (SBF).

- Until order number (8), the chemicals (**Table 2**) were added to the distilled water one at a time, after the full dissolution of each reagent.
- To prevent a local pH rise in the solution, the addition of reagent (9) should be done gradually and with less than 1gm.
- Following the addition of order number (9), the solution's temperature is examined, and pH is determined with the temperature at 37.4°C.
- The pH of the solution should be roughly identical at this value (7.5).
- To set the pH at 7.4, an HCl solution was titrated using a pipette.
- Following pH correction, 50 ml of distilled water was added to the solution, bringing its total volume to 1000 ml.
- Rinse a 1000 ml polyethylene (or polystyrene) container at least three times with a small amount of the prepared solution (SBF).
- Transfer the solution to the plastic bottle from the flask.
- The bottle was kept in a 5–10°C refrigerator.

3.2 The soaking of the samples in (SBF)

By soaking in 50 ml of Kokubo's (SBF), (**Figure 11**), the *in vitro* bioactivity of bioglass (BG), bioglass/chitosan (BG/CH), and different ratios of BG/CH dexamethasone was examined. The SBF solution has a buffered pH of (7.4) [40].

The samples in plastic containers were kept at a constant temperature of 37°C for 33 days in a thermodynamic (shaking-water bath) (see **Figure 12**).

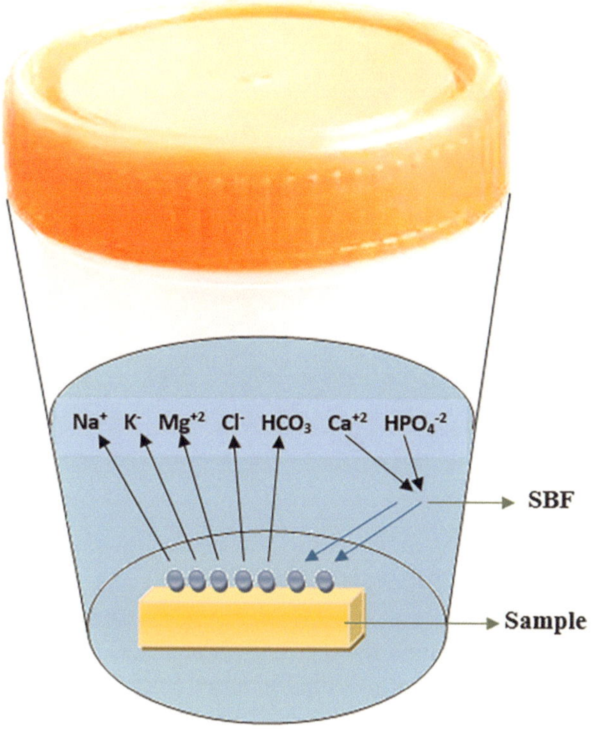

Figure 11.
Test of the static SBF in a plastic container at 37°C.

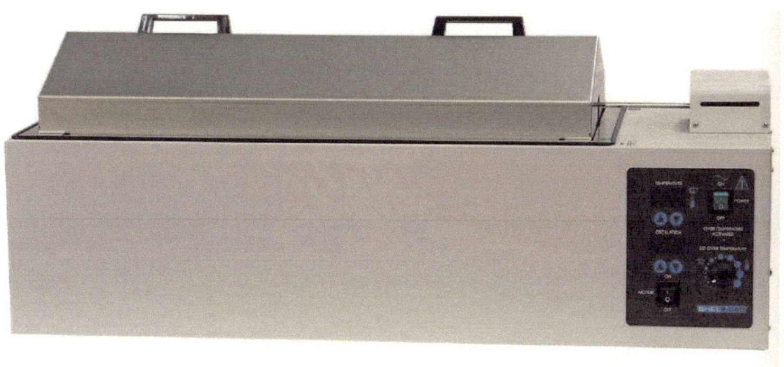

Figure 12.
Thermodynamic incubator (water bath).

The specimens were taken out of the solution, cleaned with distilled water, and then allowed to dry at room temperature after 33 days of immersion.

3.3 Elemental analysis: UV spectrophotometer technique

Each test tube had a 2 ml sample of SBF removed from it 1, 2, 4, 8, 16, 21, and 33 days after the immersion started.

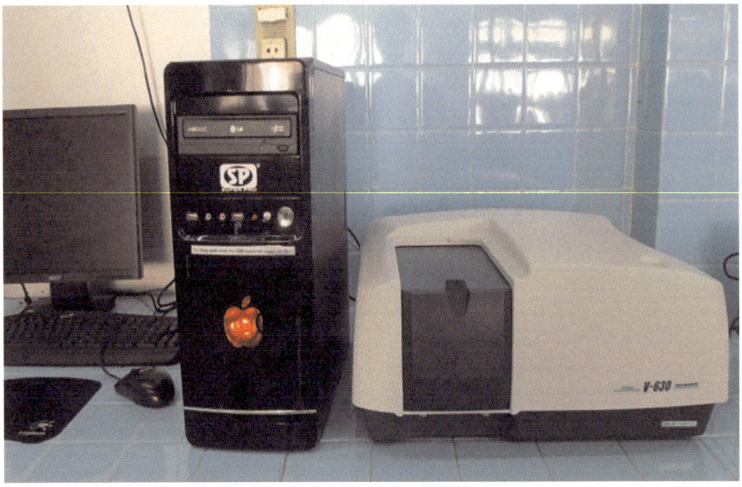

Figure 13.
UV-visible spectroscopy JASCO v-630.

And kept frozen until they were evaluated using UV-Vis spectroscopy (JASCO v-630) (see **Figure 13**) to determine the concentration of Ca, P, and dexamethasone released when a medication concentration increased over time [41].

4. Determination of drug release

4.1 Determination of the characteristic absorption peaks

The UV-visible (VIS) absorption spectra of Dexa solution are displayed in **Figure 14**. Dexa have absorption peaks were found to be strongest at wavelengths of

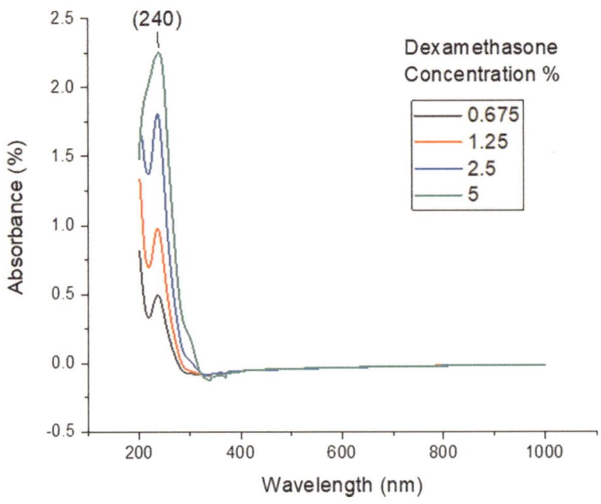

Figure 14.
UV-visible absorption spectra of dexamethasone concentration.

237, 240, and 242 nm, respectively. The absorption spectra for dexamethasone solution were photographed at 240 nm in wavelength [42].

4.2 Calibration curve of the release drug dexamethasone

Utilizing several drug reference solutions in descending order at the maximum wavelength (λ) at 240 nm, which corresponds to Dexa medicines, the UV-VIS absorption spectroscopy equipment was calibrated.

Stock solution was divided into aliquots (50, 25, 12.5, and 6.75 ml) and combined with (2 ml) of distilled water at a pH of 7.4 to create concentrations ranging from 25 to 200 g/ml. Using a UV-VIS spectrophotometer, the absorbance of these solutions was evaluated at 240 nm, as indicated in **Table 3** [43].

The drug calibration curve was altered to suit a straight line with a correlation coefficient (R^2) of 0.93692 Dexa, as shown in **Figure 15**.

no	Amount(μl)	Concentration(μg/ml)	Absorbance (%)
1	50	200	2.2532
2	25	100	1.7689
3	12.5	50	0.9557
4	6.75	25	0.4836

Table 3.
Standard absorption values of dexamethasone in distilled water pH 7.4 with different concentration.

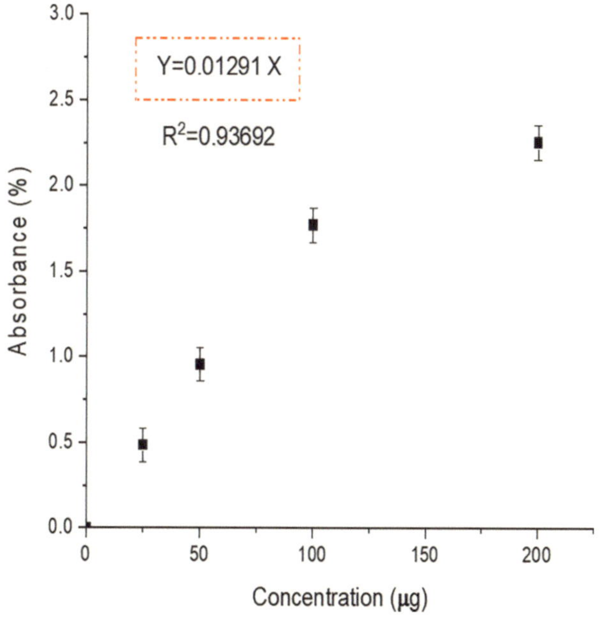

Figure 15.
Calibration curve of the release drug dexamethasone.

4.3 Determination of the amount of drug released

The dynamic *in vitro* release is depicted in **Figure 16**. Dexamethasone absorption peaks were seen in all samples individually from zero day soaking in SBF to 33 days.

UV-visible absorption spectroscopy was used to identify the absorbance peaks intensities of the drug samples across the preset time periods. The equivalent quantity of the drug was calculated using the relevant calibration curve and is shown in **Table 4** as the percentage of dexamethasone drug release.

The dexamethasone release profile revealed a lower initial release that was initially sluggish and subsequently increased. After 96 hours (4 days), the rate of Dexa release rose briefly before returning to normal (**Figure 17**).

The drug's release profile was evaluated in three stages: an initial burst release (stage I), continuous release (stage II), and declining release (stage III) (stage III).

The quantity of medication released from BG15D, BG/CH5D, BG/CH10D, and BG/CH15D composites reduced after 21 days. The profile is generally comparable for the three concentrations BG/CH5D, BG/CH10D, and BG/CH15D, as predicted given the bioglass/chitosan composites that support the medication.

The drug release is regulated by two factors: diffusion and polymer breakdown. According to the release profiles, the mechanism of Dexa release appears to be

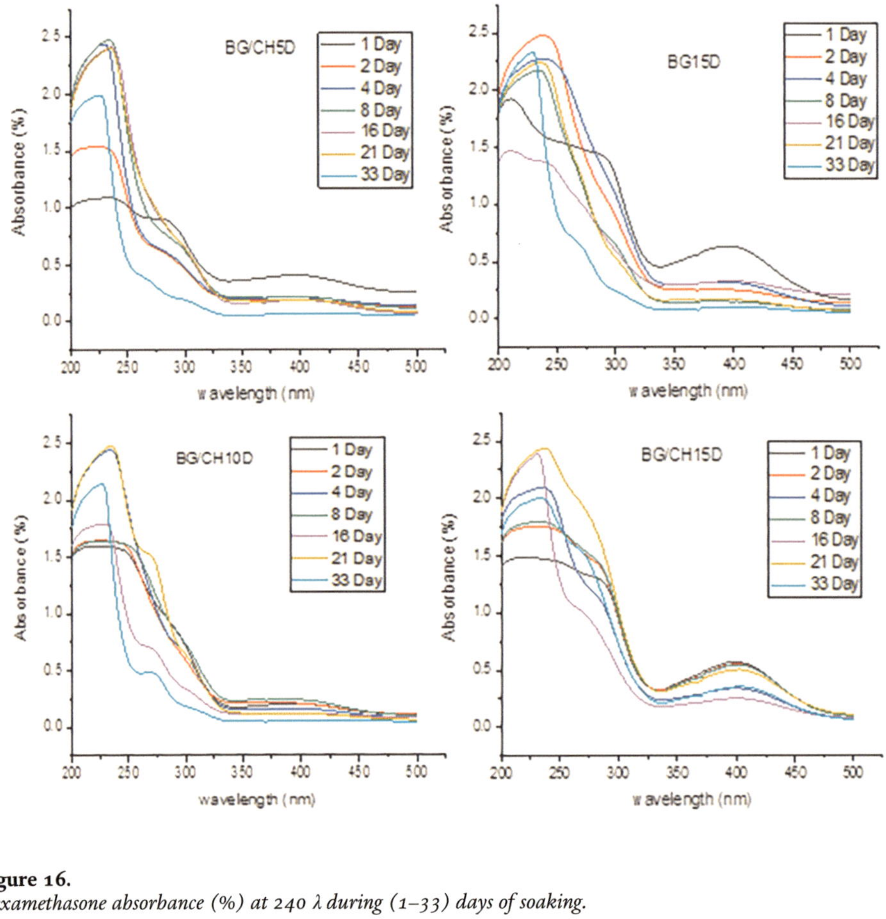

Figure 16.
Dexamethasone absorbance (%) at 240 λ during (1–33) days of soaking.

Sample Time	BG/CH5D		BG/CH10D		BG/CH15D		BG15D	
	μl	%	μl	%	μl	%	μl	%
1 day	21.05	7.73	30.77	10.88	28.57	10.24	31.64	10.85
2 days	29.50	18.58	31.80	22.14	33.93	22.40	47.87	27.279
4 days	46.41	35.63	47.32	38.88	40.55	36.93	44.01	42.37
8 days	48.00	53.28	46.45	55.32	44.47	52.87	42.11	56.82
16 days	46.61	70.41	45.64	71.47	45.64	69.22	42.16	71.28
21 days	46.41	87.46	47.94	88.44	47.09	86.10	43.33	86.15
33 days	34.09	100	32.66	100	38.77	100	40.36	100
Total amount	272.121		282.622		279.0668		291.5054	
P-value	0.01		0.01		0.01		0.01	

Table 4 shows all the percentages of dexamethasone released from all samples BG/CH5D BG/CH10D BG/CH15D BG15D and over the different periods after 1, 2, 4, 8, 16, 21 and 33 days, and it also shows the release rate of each quantity of the used drug "Dexamethasone" for each sample over the same period as previously described.

Table 4.
The percentage of dexamethasone drug released from composite samples.

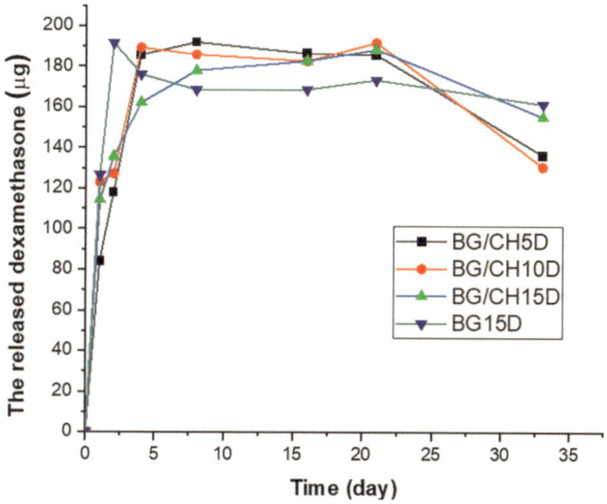

Figure 17.
The amount of release Dexa concentration from samples for (1–33) days.

through polymer breakdown rather than diffusion owing to chemical interaction amino groups of chitosan and carbonyl groups of Dexa [44].

4.4 Accumulative release of Dexa

The experimental findings showed that dexamethasone was released faster from bioglass (BG15D) than from bioglass/chitosan composites (BG/CH15D). This is owing to the fact that drug release from bioglass (BG15D) can only be impacted by diffusion, but drug release from BG/CH5D, BG/CH10D, and BG/CH15D may be sustained by chitosan degradation based on the chemical interaction of chitosan amino groups and dexamethasone carbonyl groups (**Figure 18**).

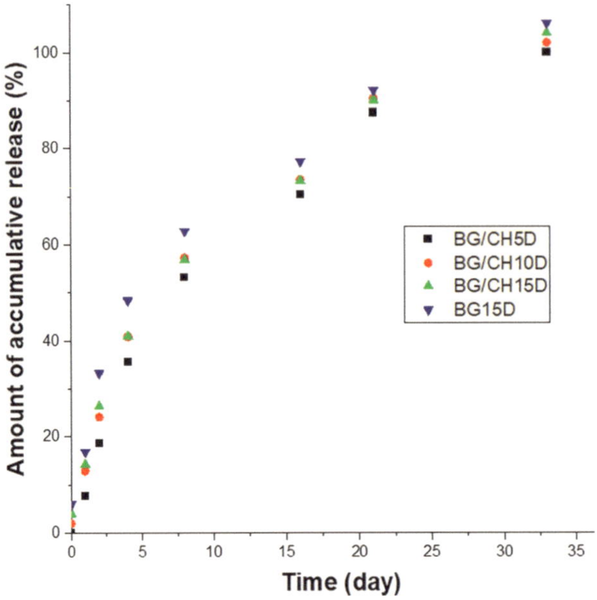

Figure 18.
Release profile of dexamethasone in terms of the percentage (%) of dexamethasone released as a function of time.

5. Conclusion

At various dilution ratios, the controlled release was tested using "JASCO v-630" UV visible spectroscopy. A standard curve was developed to establish a link between the absorption rate, as measured by the UV device, and the drug concentration in the medium utilized (SBF). The release profile reveals that the dexamethasone release may be sustained for more than 30 days, and the drug release experimental data indicate that the release is driven by chitosan polymer breakdown. Based on the findings of this study, we can conclude that (bioglass/chitosan) is a good function material as a carrier for anti-inflammatory dexamethasone drug as a corticosteroid and that it may be successfully employed in bone tissue engineering applications.

It has been determined that the release profile showed that the dexamethasone release may be sustained for more than 30 days, and the drug release experimental data indicate that the release is driven by chitosan polymer breakdown. Based on the findings of this investigation, we therefore proposed that bioglass/chitosan is a suitable functional material as a carrier for the anti-inflammatory medication dexamethasone in this study.

Acknowledgements

I first and foremost thank the All-Powerful Allah for both my possessions and lack of possessions. He is the ruler of the universe. Salutations to Muhammad (PBUH), the finest and most excellent of all beings. Among the academics I am grateful to and indebted to are my brother Dr. Ahmed Ali Abdel-Aal Mohamed, my best friend Dr. Abd elrahmaan Al-esnawy, and my teachers Dr. Ahmed S. Abd raboh, Prof. Dr. M. Y. Hassan, and Prof. Dr. Khairy M. T. Ereiba of the Faculty of Science at Al-Azhar University.

Conflict of interest

Not applicable.

Author details

Mohamed S. El-Khooly[1,2]

1 Faculty of Science, Biophysics Branch, Physics Department, Al-Azhar University, Nasr City, Cairo, Egypt

2 Faculty of Science, Physics Department, New Valley University, El Kharga, New Valley, Egypt

*Address all correspondence to: ms.new39@gmail.com

References

[1] Green D, Walsh D, Yang X, Mann S, Oreffo ROC. Stimulation of human bone marrow stromal cells using growth factor encapsulated calcium carbonate porous microspheres. Journal of Materials Chemistry. 2004;**14**(14):2206-2212. DOI: 10.1039/b400486h

[2] Eroğlu H et al. The in-vitro and in-vivo characterization of PLGA:L-PLA microspheres containing dexamethasone sodium phosphate. Journal of Microencapsulation. 2001;**18**(5):603-612. DOI: 10.1080/02652040010019587

[3] Yoon JJ, Kim JH, Park TG. Dexamethasone-releasing biodegradable polymer scaffolds fabricated by a gas-foaming/salt-leaching method. Biomaterials. 2003;**24**(13):2323-2329. DOI: 10.1016/S0142-9612(03)00024-3

[4] Gomes ME, Reis RL. Biodegradable polymers and composites in biomedical applications: From catgut to tissue engineering part 1 available systems and their properties. International Materials Review. 2004;**49**(5): 261-273. DOI: 10.1179/095066004225021918

[5] James JE. Symptoms of alcoholism in women: A preliminary survey of A.A. members. Journal of Studies on Alcohol. 1975;**36**(11):1564-1569

[6] Habraken WJEM, Wolke JGC, Jansen JA. Ceramic composites as matrices and scaffolds for drug delivery in tissue engineering. Advanced Drug Delivery Reviews. 2007;**59**(4–5): 234-248. DOI: 10.1016/j.addr.2007.03.011

[7] Raboh ASA, El-khooly MS, Hassaan MY. Bioactivity and drug release study of dexamethasone loaded bioglass/chitosan composites for biomedical applications. Journal of Inorganic and Organometallic Polymers and Materials. 2021;**31**(7):2779-2790. DOI: 10.1007/s10904-021-01936-z

[8] Siepmann J, Siegel RA, Rathbone MJ. Fundamentals and applications of controlled release drug delivery. In: *Fundamentals and Application of Controlled Release Drug Delivery*. New York, NY: Springer; 2012. pp. 1-594. DOI: 10.1007/978-1-4614-0881-9

[9] Reddy LH, Bazile D. Drug delivery design for intravenous route with integrated physicochemistry, pharmacokinetics and pharmacodynamics: Illustration with the case of taxane therapeutics. Advanced Drug Delivery Reviews. 2014;**71**(2013):34-57. DOI: 10.1016/j.addr.2013.10.007

[10] Tiwari G et al. Drug delivery systems: An updated review. International Journal of Pharmaceutical Investigation. 2012;**2**(1):2. DOI: 10.4103/2230-973x.96920

[11] Lee JH, Yeo Y. Controlled drug release from pharmaceutical nanocarriers. Chemical Engineering Science. 2015;**125**:75-84. DOI: 10.1016/j.ces.2014.08.046

[12] Lee PI, Li JX. Evolution of oral controlled release dosage forms. In: Oral Controlled Release Formulation Design and Drug Delivery Theory to Practice. New Jersey: Wiley; 2010. pp. 21-31. DOI: 10.1002/9780470640487.ch2

[13] Fisk P. Creative genius: An innovation guide for business leaders, border crossers and game changers. United Kingdom. 2007;**46**(40): 7519-7713. Available from: https://online

library.wiley.com/doi/10.1002/anie.200604488

[14] Tomei AA, Villa C, Ricordi C. Development of an encapsulated stem cell-based therapy for diabetes. Expert Opinion on Biological Therapy. 2015;**15**(9):1321-1336. DOI: 10.1517/14712598.2015.1055242

[15] Yun YH, Lee BK, Park K. Controlled drug delivery: Historical perspective for the next generation. Journal of Controlled Release. 2015;**219**:2-7. DOI: 10.1016/j.jconrel.2015.10.005

[16] Vallet-Regí M, Arcos D. Bioceramics for drug delivery. Acta Materialia. 2013;**61**(3):890-911. DOI: 10.1016/j.actamat.2012.10.039

[17] Olsen TW et al. Cannulation of the Suprachoroidal space: A novel drug delivery methodology to the posterior segment. American Journal of Ophthalmology. 2006;**142**(5):777-787.e2

[18] Hornig S, Bunjes H, Heinze T. Preparation and characterization of nanoparticles based on dextran-drug conjugates. Journal of Colloid and Interface Science. 2009;**338**(1):56-62. DOI: 10.1016/j.jcis.2009.05.025

[19] Ta HT, Dass CR, Dunstan DE. Injectable chitosan hydrogels for localised cancer therapy. Journal of Controlled Release. 2008;**126**(3):205-216. DOI: 10.1016/j.jconrel.2007.11.018

[20] Ramakrishna S, Mayer J, Wintermantel E, Leong KW. Biomedical applications of polymer-composite materials: A review. Composites Science and Technology. 2001;**61**(9):1189-1224. DOI: 10.1016/S0266-3538(00)00241-4

[21] Nathan AJ, Scobell A. How China sees America. Foreign Affairs. 2012;**91**(5)

[22] Vallet-Regí M, Balas F, Arcos D. Mesoporous materials for drug delivery. Angewandte Chemie – International Edition. 2007;**46**(40):7548-7558. DOI: 10.1002/anie.200604488

[23] Kaur G. Clinical applications of biomaterials: State-of-the-art progress, trends, and novel approaches. In: Clinical Applications of Biomaterials. State-of-the-Art Progress, Trends, and Novel Approaches. Cham: Springer; 2017. pp. 1-467. DOI: 10.1007/978-3-319-56059-5

[24] Ding H et al. A novel injectable borate bioactive glass cement as an antibiotic delivery vehicle for treating osteomyelitis. PLoS One. 2014;**9**(1):1-9. DOI: 10.1371/journal.pone.0085472

[25] Haran-Ghera N, Peled A, Krautghamer R, Resnitzky P. Initiation and promotion in radiation-induced myeloid leukemia. Leukemia. 1992;**6**(7):689-695 Available from: http://europepmc.org/abstract/MED/1625487

[26] Ma J et al. Hierarchical porous bioactive glasses/PLGA-magnetic SBA-15 for dual-drug release. Materials Science and Engineering: C. 2014;**39**(1):21-28. DOI: 10.1016/j.msec.2014.01.060

[27] Montani D, Seferian A, Savale L, Simonneau G, Humbert M. Drug-induced pulmonary arterial hypertension: A recent outbreak. European Respiratory Review. 2013;**22**(129):244-250. DOI: 10.1183/09059180.00003313

[28] Al-Idrissi HY, Ibrahim EM, Abdullah KA, Ababtain WA, Boukhary HA, Macaulay HMK. Antiemetic efficacy of high-dose dexamethasone: Randomized, double-blind, crossover study with a combination of dexamethasone, metoclopramide and diphenhydramine.

British Journal of Cancer. 1988;**57**(3): 308-312. DOI: 10.1038/bjc.1988.68

[29] Wang H, Li M, Rinehart JJ, Zhang R. Pretreatment with dexamethasone increases antitumor activity of carboplatin and gemcitabine in mice bearing human cancer xenografts: In vivo activity, pharmacokinetics, and clinical implications for cancer chemotherapy. Clinical Cancer Research. 2004;**10**(5):1633-1644. DOI: 10.1158/ 1078-0432.CCR-0829-3

[30] Calignano A, Persico P, Mancuso F, Sorrentino L. Adenosine release in morphine-induced hypotension in rats. General Pharmacology. 1992;**23**(1):7-10. DOI: 10.1016/0306-3623(92)90039-M

[31] Senior HEJ et al. Supported living service assessment. Journal of the American Medical Directors Association. 2014;**22**(6):588-597. Available from: h ttps://onlinelibrary.wiley.com/doi/full/ 10.1111/hsc.12105

[32] F. Regulations. Parallel table of authorities and rules. [Online]. 899–1014. 2016. Available from: http://www.ecfr.gov/cgi-bin/ECFR?page=browse

[33] Thomas S, Perry SF. Control and consequences of adrenergic activation of red blood cell Na+/H+ exchange on blood oxygen and carbon dioxide transport in fish. The Journal of Experimental Zoology. 1992;**263**(2): 160-175. DOI: 10.1002/jez.1402630206

[34] BUDAVARI S. An Encyclopedia of chemicals, drugs, and biologicals. The Merck Index. 1989;**246** Available from: https://ci.nii.ac.jp/naid/10003733334/en/

[35] Howard M. Evaluation of the physicochemical properties and stability of solid lipid nanoparticles designed for the delivery of dexamethasone to. University of Kentucky, 2011. pp.1-276. Available from: https://uknowledge.uky.edu/gradschool_diss/806M. Howard, Evaluation of the physicochemical properties and stability of solid lipid nanoparticles designed for the delivery of dexamethasone to, 1–30, 2011.

[36] Chen M, Vijay V, Shi Q, Liu Z, Fang H, Tong W. FDA-approved drug labeling for the study of drug-induced liver injury. Drug Discovery Today. 2011;**6**(15–16):697-703. DOI: 10.1016/ j.drudis.2011.05.007

[37] Malet G, Munoz F, Appleyard R, Hersh W. A model for enhancing internet medical document retrieval with 'medical core metadata'. Journal of the American Medical Informatics Association. 1999;**6**(2):163-172. DOI: 10.1136/jamia.1999.0060163

[38] Cohen V, Jellinek SP, Teperikidis L, Berkovits E, Goldman WM. Room-temperature storage of medications labeled for refrigeration. American Journal of Health-System Pharmacy. 2007;**64**(16):1711-1715. DOI: 10.2146/ ajhp060262

[39] Kokubo T, Takadama H. How useful is SBF in predicting in vivo bone bioactivity? Biomaterials. 2006;**27**(15): 2907-2915. DOI: 10.1016/j.biomaterials. 2006.01.017

[40] Al-esnawy AA, Ereiba KT, Bakr AM, Abdraboh AS. Characterization and antibacterial activity of streptomycin Sulfate loaded bioglass/chitosan beads for bone tissue engineering. Journal of Molecular Structure. 2021;**1227**:129715. DOI: 10.1016/j.molstruc.2020.129715

[41] El-khooly MS, Abdraboh AS, Bakr AM, Ereiba KHT. Bioactivity and mechanical properties characterization of bioactive glass incorporated with graphene oxide. SILICON. 2022:

0123456789. DOI: 10.1007/s12633-022-02088-6

[42] Forteza M, Galán E, Cornejo J. Interaction of dexamethasone and montmorillonite - adsorption-degradation process. Applied Clay Science. 1989;**4**(5–6):437-448. DOI: 10.1016/0169-1317(89)90021-5

[43] Gandhimathi C. Controlled release of dexamethasone in PCL/silk fibroin/ ascorbic acid nanoparticles for the initiation of adipose derived stem cells into osteogenesis. Journal of Drug Metabolism & Toxicology. 2015;**06**(02): 1-7. DOI: 10.4172/2157-7609.1000177

[44] Chiang ZC, Yu SH, Chao AC, Dong GC. Preparation and characterization of dexamethasone-immobilized chitosan scaffold. Journal of Bioscience and Bioengineering. 2012; **113**(5):654-660. DOI: 10.1016/j.jbiosc.2012.01.002

Section 2

Safety and Consequences Related to Corticosteroids Use

Chapter 5

Safe Use of Cortisol for Inflammation Disorders

Virgil I. Stenberg and Ann L. Baldwin

Abstract

In 1992, the hypothalamus-pituitary-adrenal (HPA) axis was proposed to be the inflammation control system of the body. The cortisol pulse that emanates from this axis when activated is the inflammation gatekeeper that terminates short-term, beneficial inflammation at is due time. As the cortisol pulse weakens with age, injury and heredity, the termination becomes incomplete. Then, the residual short-term inflammation evolves into long-term, destructive inflammation within inflammation disorders. In support of the proposal, induced inflammation in normal rats causes a corticosterone pulse. If the proposal were correct, the inflammation disease solution would be to supplement the cortisol pulse at the proper time. Twenty-one (21) participants with rheumatoid arthritis entered a double-blind, crossover study using patient self-administered prednisone. The 18 completing the study averaged a record 75% symptom improvement with no significant side effects. Further, 2428 participants with 38 inflammation disorders entered an open study using patient self-administrated cortisol. The 2015 completing the study averaged 76% symptom improvement with no significant side effects.

Keywords: cortisol, hydrocortisone, cortisol pulse, prednisone, hypothalamus-pituitary-adrenal axis, inflammation, inflammatory diseases, inflammation diseases, rheumatoid arthritis

1. Introduction

Excellent cortisone studies that have been published after the Nobel Prize work of Hench, Kendal, and Reichstein [1, 2] are sufficient to resolve the cortisone controversy and solve arthritis. Our confidence in so doing, gained by achieving an average 75% symptom improvement in multiple arthritis diseases, emboldens us to expose our base concepts. You must decide if we are correct. Life restoration for millions lie in the balance.

2. Colorful cortisone: first demonstration arthritis is solvable

Hench had guessed the adrenal glands are producing a hormone that would reverse arthritis. In 1948, Sarett synthesized a candidate chemical, cortisone, identified from among the many steroids made by the adrenal glands [3–5]. At the 1949 meeting of the

American College of Rheumatology, Hench presented before and after movies of the arthritics being treated with cortisone. Hench received a standing ovation. In 1950, he was awarded the Nobel Prize. The price of cortisone became 100 times that of gold.

3. The dilemma

When cortisone was administered in dosages sufficient to arrest arthritis, prohibitive side effects occurred. When the dosages were lowered to where the side effects did not occur, arthritis remained.

4. The 1960 cortisone decision

A fateful decision was made about 1960 that cortisone in tablet form is unsafe except for short-term use to resolve inflammation crises in patients but safe when given by injections. In 2022, doctors of medicine remained reluctant to prescribe cortisol tablets for people with inflammation diseases even within the safe use limits [6]. Those who dare violate the decision risk being disciplined by state boards of examiners. We, as research scientists concentrating on cortisone, have been requested to appear before two boards of medical examiners in two states though we are beyond their jurisdiction.

5. The 1960 decision is theoretically incorrect

Cortisone, as a hormone made by the body, cannot have side effects at least within physiological concentrations. If it did, all people would exhibit cortisol side effects. The safe limits of cortisone use have been defined [6]. The perceived side effects most probably occur from administering cortisone beyond its safe use limits through lack of understanding. The 1960 decision contributes to the cortisone controversy.

6. Eliminating perceived side effects

The 1960 decision has dominated cortisone use in clinic practice for the past 6 decades. Doctors of medicine tried different ways of administering cortisone to retain its wonderful efficacy for arresting arthritis while avoiding its perceived side effects: daily use, alternate day use, bolus therapy, and pulse therapy. The results were unsatisfactory.

Chemists synthesized near-similar cortisone molecules that would retain its arthritis efficacy yet eliminate its perceived side effects [7]. From this, prednisone, prednisolone, methylprednisolone, dexamethasone, betamethasone, and triamcinolone became commercially available. These synthetics failed to eliminate cortisone's perceived side effects.

7. 1960 to present

Although this chapter focuses upon cortisone and arthritis, the significant contribution of non-cortisone research must be acknowledged. Of these, adalimumab leads by achieving 41–61% symptom improvement for rheumatoid arthritis. Of the cortisone family, patient self-administration of cortisol with stress management leads by achieving an average 76% symptom improvement with no significant adverse reactions [8].

8. Cortisone

By the 1960 decision, cortisone in tablet form has been and is being denied a prominent role in long-term care of arthritis. The dream of somehow using cortisone for long-term care of arthritis patients remains alive [1, 2]. It is tempting to discard cortisone as a word for it is a minor component of the adrenal exudate and inactive for treating arthritis. For it to become active, it must first be converted by the body into cortisol.

However, cortisone continues to maintain universal interest. The word cortisone has been born into all languages. Currently, the word cortisone has grown to represent any one of cortisol and its synthetics. It would be impractical to discard the word cortisone for its broader definition is useful. Nevertheless, the word cortisone has been and is contributing to the cortisone controversy.

9. Cortisol

Cortisol is the only body-made chemical that perfectly arrests the out-of-control inflammation within arthritis. It is continuously produced by the two adrenal glands at the combined rate of approximately 20 mg each 24 hours. It possesses a high lethal dose, a low overdose level that causes Cushing syndrome, and an adrenal suppression ability when administered improperly.

Cortisol is essential for maintaining homeostasis. Below its normal concentration range in the body, Addison's disease threatens. Cortisol is defined to be a stress hormone. The body produces more during periods of stress. Cortisol could as well be defined as the inflammation hormone for it is also produced more after an inflammation insult to the body. It reverses the vascular swelling and porosity induced by inflammation.

Cortisol is correctly defined to be a steroid. The base chemical structure of cortisol is indeed the steroid chassis. However, other hormones and plant chemicals are built upon this chemical chassis as well. Such chemicals include cholesterol, estrogen, progesterone, testosterone, and estrogen. Using the word steroid to represent cortisol and its synthetics is incorrect and contributes to the cortisone controversy.

Hydrocortisone is a second name for cortisol of equal usage rate. Cortisol is employed when its role as a hormone is the subject. Hydrocortisone is employed when its role as an administered medicine is the subject. This dual nomenclature for the same chemical that attributes its perceived side effects to hydrocortisone and hormonal effects to cortisol is incorrect, unnecessary, confusing, and contributes to the cortisone controversy.

Glucocorticoid is a third name for cortisol or one of its synthetics. The name implies a chemical in the adrenal cortex exudate that induces increased glucose in the blood. Cortisol's synthetics are not in the adrenal cortex exudate. Consequently, the term glucocorticoid is incorrectly used, unnecessary, too nonspecific, and contributes to the cortisone controversy.

Corticosteroid is a fourth name for cortisol or one of its synthetics. The term means all chemicals in the adrenal exudate that have a steroid chassis. The cortisol synthetics are not in the adrenal exudate. Other steroids than cortisone and cortisol in the adrenal exudate do not have the hormonal properties of cortisol. Consequently, the term corticosteroids is too specific, incorrect as used, and contributes to the cortisone controversy.

10. Cortisone controversy and arthritis

The cortisone controversy would be a non-entity were it not for the titillation that somehow cortisone is the solution for arthritis.

11. Arthritis

Arthritis is ravaging citizens of all countries regardless of stature or wealth.

Arthritis is dictionary-defined to be inflammation in the body joints. In use, its definition has grown to represent out-of-control inflammation in any part of the body. Subcategories of the arthritis have been given specific names such as carditis for heart inflammation and pancreatitis for pancreas inflammation. When the inflammation resides at multiple body sites simultaneously, names such as fibromyalgia, rheumatoid arthritis, and osteoarthritis are invoked. Altogether, these compose the arthritis family of diseases.

The time-honored way of identifying a disease with a name by similar symptom grouping fails when applied to out-of-control inflammation. There are an infinite number of combinations of body areas wherein out-of-control inflammation can reside. These inflammation sites can and do change with time. To apply names based on symptom grouping is like chasing the wind.

The arthritis family of diseases is a subcategory of inflammatory diseases or more properly inflammation diseases. Within the latter, diseases caused by inflammation in the brain and lungs must also be included such as Parkinson's disease, multiple sclerosis, neuropathy, and asthma. The borderline between inflammation diseases and non-inflammation diseases is incompletely defined. Naming of inflammation diseases by similar symptoms contributes to the cortisone controversy.

12. Inflammation

Inflammation is the common denominator of inflammation diseases. Injuries, allergies, and infections are the causes of inflammation. Inflammation manifestations are heat, redness, swelling, and pain. After an inflammation cause initiates inflammation at a site, the blood vessels of the site increase in diameter and porosity. The increased porosity allows pressurized plasma in the blood to exit forming rivers and lakes within the inflammation site. The increased porosity also allows immune cells, normally constrained to the blood, to exit the blood vessels and migrate to all areas of the inflammation site via the plasma lakes and rivers to perform their tasks.

13. Inflammation vs. cortisol-responding diseases

There is no difference between inflammation diseases and cortisol-responding diseases.

14. Inflammation diseases vs. autoimmune diseases

Autoimmune diseases can be considered to be a subcategory of inflammation diseases. If an inflammation were to last beyond it due time, the continuous flow of immune cells into the inflammation site would give the appearance of an autoimmune response. Immune cells accumulate within the swollen tissues of the inflammation site. Older immune cells walls rupture to release indiscriminate enzymes that dismantle normal body tissue to create destruction.

Inflammation is an essential prerequisite to the immune response in inflammation diseases. If out-of-control inflammation were to be perfectly arrested, the autoimmune response would be simultaneously arrested.

The autoimmune response is site specific. If it were to occur simultaneously throughout the body, the body would likely not survive. The term autoimmune disease should be discontinued. The autoimmune concept is misleading, unnecessary, and contributes to the cortisone controversy.

15. Out-of-control inflammation vs. arthritis

Once the out-of-control inflammation within inflammation diseases is perfectly arrested, there is nothing left but damage done. By analogy, it is like pricking an inflated balloon to leave behind the elastic remnants of the inflated balloon. Therefore, inflammation diseases, as we know them, are but one: out-of-control inflammation disease. Each of the hitherto arthritis diseases differ only by the various locations of inflammation within the body. Some of the arthritis diseases are amalgams of inflammation in multiple locations [9].

16. Inflammation control system

The inflammation within out-of-control inflammation is identical to that within short-term, beneficial inflammation in all but lifetimes. Therefore, the body must have an inflammation control system that terminates short-term, beneficial inflammation at its due time to prevent it from evolving into long-term, destructive inflammation. With this hypothetical inflammation control system, short-term, beneficial inflammation is arrested at its due time. This system must have an on-demand feature since inflammation occurrences are irregular and unpredictable. The system must employ cortisol as the terminating agent because it is the only option.

17. Inflammation control system identified

The hypothalamus-pituitary-adrenal (HPA) axis fulfills both requirements for being the inflammation control system of the body. The on-demand activation feature of the axis responds as need to the irregular timing of inflammation initiation. After activation, the axis emits a short-term, huge, 6 + fold concentration, time-delayed cortisol pulse into the blood. The purpose of this cortisol pulse presumably is to arrest short-term, beneficial inflammation at its due time. The HPA axis, long regarded as an important intellectual curiosity, is thus elevated to be one of the most important regulatory systems of the body – the inflammation control system that prevents inflammation diseases.

18. Cause of inflammation disease

The hypothesis for the cause of inflammation disease is the cortisol pulse emanating from the HPA-axis activated by stress weakens with age, heredity or injury to make the body vulnerable to any source of inflammation. It will be unable to adequately quench short-term inflammation at its due time thereby allowing long-term, destructive inflammation within inflammation disease to evolve.

To prove the correctness of this hypothesis in the laboratory, non-diseased, normal rats were injected with an inflammatory agent to initiate inflammation [10]. Hours later, the rat's equivalent of human cortisol, corticosterone, concentration peaked in its blood at 12x of its restive state concentration. Thereafter, its concentration receded to the restive state concentration again. Thereby, connection between initiated inflammation and the corticosterone pulse in rats is established. The connection between initiated inflammation and the cortisol pulse in humans is inferred.

When non-diseased, normal rats, surgically altered to prevent them from making the natural corticosterone pulse, were injected with the same inflammatory agent, the rats gained the appearance of arthritis with slow movements and squealing from pain. Therefore, the corticosterone pulse can be assumed to be the controlling agent that prevents normal rats from gaining the appearance of arthritis in the first experiment.

The rat experiment results are consistent with the hypothesis illustrated in **Figure 1**.

19. Adrenal glands produce cortisol in two ways

The adrenal glands maintain the normal level of cortisol in the blood at all times – a little more in the morning and a little less in the evening to constitute its diurnal rhythm. The adrenal glands also supply the cortisol on demand to enable the HPA-axis to make its inflammation-induced cortisol pulse. As adrenal cortisol output weakens with age, injury, and heredity, the first to weaken is HPA-axis cortisol pulse that allows inflammation diseases. As adrenal cortisol output weakens further, inflammation and Addison's diseases threaten, cf. **Figure 2**.

20. Laboratory unable to detect cortisol pulse weakening

Routine laboratory analysis for cortisol concentration in patients with inflammation disease will detect no difference from normal concentrations of cortisol in the blood. This is because laboratory analyses will most probably occur during non-flare times of the body. The results have been and should be within the normal range. If the laboratory analysis occurs during times of inflammation, the laboratory results

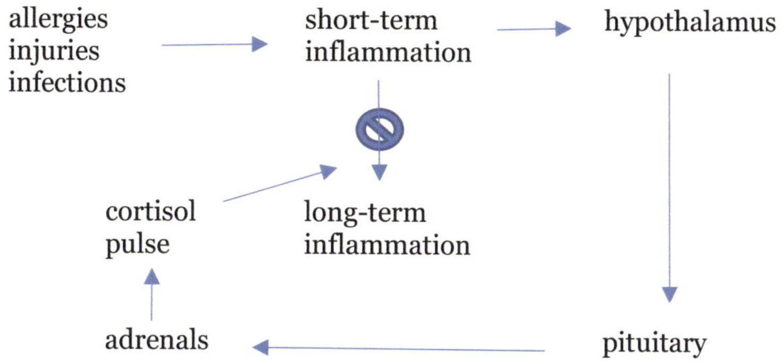

Figure 1.
The inflammation control system of the body. Short-term inflammation, caused by one of the three sources of inflammation, activates the HPA-axis to produce a time-delayed cortisol pulse. This pulse prevents short-term inflammation from evolving into the long-term inflammation within inflammation disease.

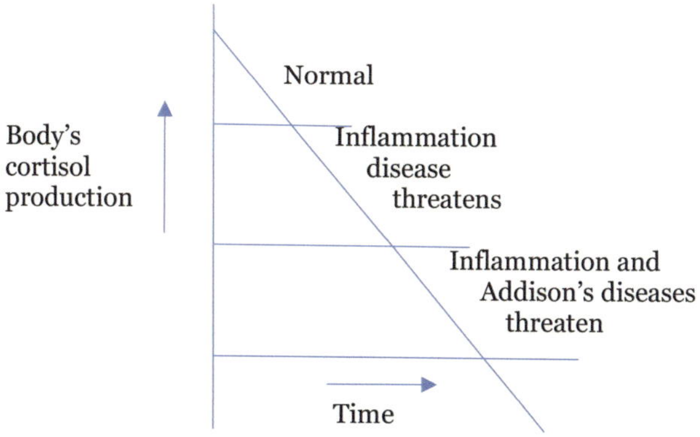

Figure 2.
Inflammation disease threatens when the body's cortisol production deteriorates to where the cortisol pulse weakens. Inflammation and Addison's diseases threaten when the adrenal cortisol output deteriorates further.

will either be within the normal range in the event of adrenal exhaustion or elevated if not. In any event, laboratory analysis will be unreliable for detecting weakening cortisol pulse emanating from the HPA-axis.

21. Patient self-administration of cortisol

If the weakening cortisol pulse of the HPA-axis is the cause of out-of-control inflammation within inflammation disease, then restoring the weakening pulse to its optimum size will be the solution. The pulse restoration must begin promptly when short-term, beneficial inflammation begins to evolve into long-term, destructive inflammation. At this time, patients will experience increases in pain, fatigue, and movement restriction, i.e., a flare. Since only patients will know when a flare is in progress, patient self-administration of cortisol is required for the solution.

The amount of cortisol to arrest each flare and number of consecutive days to complete the arrest had to be empirically determined. From pretrial rheumatoid arthritis patients, these were 5 days and 25 mg prednisone (100 mg cortisol), respectively. These data are contingent upon identifying and promptly treating each flare in its earliest stage. As the flare intensity increased, more cortisol was required.

The distribution of the cortisol amount per flare over the 5 days had to be empirically determined. From pretrial rheumatoid arthritis patients, this was established to be 7.5 mg prednisone (30 mg cortisol) per day for day 1, 5 mg prednisone (20 mg cortisol) per day for days 2–4, and 2.5 mg prednisone (10 mg cortisol) for day 5. Tapering was recommended by physician counselors and not from theory. The average flare frequency of occurrence had to be empirically determined. Its determination had to await the first clinical trial.

22. Double-blind human trial

Twenty-one (21) people with rheumatoid arthritis volunteered to participate in a double-blind crossover clinical trial to determine the effectiveness of patient self-administration of prednisone. Eighteen (18) patients completed the protocol to average a record 75% symptom improvement [11]. The average rheumatoid arthritis flares per month was 3.3.

The 2428-participant open study.

When patient self-administration of cortisol with stress management was applied to 2428 patients with 38 chronic inflammation diseases, symptom improvement exceeded that of standard treatments two-fold [8]. The treatment efficacies and response rates were the same within experimental error for the diseases of the study. When patients used cortisol tablets for pulse restoration on the bad days and not on the good days (as short-term, beneficial is evolving into long-term, destructive inflammation), so little cortisol was ingested that overdose adverse effects were avoided. Only the missing cortisol was being replaced. The average daily consumption of cortisol using patient self-administration was 12 mg per day. This is less than the minimum 15 mg daily cortisol use that causes overdose symptoms in the most sensitive patients [3]. Consequently, the name patient self-administration of cortisol with stress management was shortened to microcortisol therapy since patient's average using less cortisol per day is than the 20 to 52 mg per day dose range of low-dose cortisol.

23. Patient self-administration of cortisol with stress management

Patient self-administration of cortisol alone can fail to give satisfactory effectiveness when an active source of inflammation or an inflammation exacerbation source is present. Of injuries, infections [12], allergies [13], and emotional traumas (an exacerbation source), the last three are most frequent. Patients handle injuries including overexercise without assistance.

Patients are unaware that occult infections cause inflammation that counteracts the beneficial effects of cortisol. Those who fail to achieve about 75 + % symptom improvement during the initial phase of the protocol take a broad-spectrum antibiotic for a sufficient period of time to determine if another significant improvement can be made. Doxycycline taken in the normal adult dosage for 1–2 months is a favorite.

Patients are unaware food allergies can cause inflammation that counteracts the beneficial effects of cortisol. Allergy responses cause inflammation. When partial but imperfect control of an inflammation disease is achieved by patient self-administration of cortisol alone, patients should search for allergenic foods.

When patients are made aware that a food can make their out-of-control inflammation worse, they willingly cooperate to search for the culprit food or foods.

Disorder	n Efficacy	%
Fibromyalgia	601	77
Osteoarthritis	579	77
Rheumatoid arthritis	248	78
Arthritis, undifferentiated	226	76
Back pain	75	70
Parkinson's disease	51	62
Polymyalgia rheumatica	44	80
Chronic fatigue syndrome	25	78
Neuropathy	25	74
Dementia, Parkinson's disease	22	67
Headache, migraine	21	86
Multiple sclerosis	19	67
Asthma	11	68
Systemic lupus erythematosis	9	60
Bursitis	6	79
Irritable bowel syndrome	6	71
Psoriatic arthritis	6	63
Crohn's disease	5	92
Carpal tunnel syndrome	5	86
Spinal stenosis	4	78
Headache	3	84
Nervous system symptoms	3	63
Ankylosing spondylitis	3	60
Urinary tract inflammation	3	58
Post traumatic stress disorder	2	71
Acid reflux	1	100
Bowel inflammation	1	100
Scoliosis	1	100
Dementia, rheumatoid arthr	1	92
Dementia	1	86
Eye inflammation	1	85
Eczema	1	77
Myofacial syndrome	1	73
Meniere's disease	1	69
Sjogren's syndrome	1	69
Dementia, multiple sclerosis	1	67
Restless leg syndrome	1	47

Table 1.
Open study results using patient self-administration of cortisol with stress management.

Elimination diets and food allergy tests are helpful tools. Airborne allergen testing is secondary since airborne allergens would be expected to be associated with lung inflammation disease. The ultimate test is removal of the culprit food from the patient's diet and the patient gets better; restoring the food to the patient's diet and the patient gets worse.

Patients are unaware emotional traumas cause inflammation that counteracts the beneficial effects of cortisol. When partial but imperfect control of an inflammation disease is achieved by patient self-administration of cortisol alone, patients should be asked about emotional traumas in their lives. Examples of these traumas are positive ones like going on a cruise or vacation or negative ones like a divorce or bankruptcy. Emotional traumas must be minimized if not avoided for optimum success.

See **Table 1** for summary of data from the 2428-participant study.

24. Patient's response rates to cortisol differ

On patient self-administration of cortisol alone, one of 6 lost most or all symptoms in 1 week, 4 of 6 more lost the symptoms within 4 weeks, and the remaining 1 of 6 failed to respond satisfactory when employing the cortisol dosages published [8]. This factor is a major contributor to the cortisone controversy.

25. Conclusions

The hypothalamus-pituitary-adrenal (HPA) axis is the body's inflammation control system.

The cause of inflammation disease is a weakened cortisol pulse from an activated HPA axis.

The solution to inflammation disease is HPA cortisol pulse restoration.

Patient self-administration of cortisol is the optimum methodology for cortisol pulse restoration.

Patient self-administration of cortisol achieves a record average 76% symptom improvement when treating inflammation disease.

Patient self-administration of cortisol applied to inflammation disease exhibits no significant side effects.

Patient self-administration of cortisol with stress management leaves damage done.

Patients respond to cortisol administration at differing rates.

Diseases with out-of-control inflammation are but one disease – inflammation disease.

Inflammation symptoms differ by the various localized inflammation locations within the body.

Inflammation diseases are treatable by on treatment protocol.

Autoimmune diseases are a subcategory of inflammation diseases.

With the new assigned role of the PPA-axis, the cortisone controversy disappears.

Acknowledgements

Microdose therapy was created to solve Helen Stenberg's intractable rheumatoid arthritis. In 1984, she became asymptomatic using microcortisol therapy and remained as such with no significant adverse reactions until her passing from cancer in 2017. Her story is portrayed in the 1996 book entitled Arthritis. The Simple Solution available from Amazon. The contributions of the volunteer pretrial patients were essential for designing patient self-administration of cortisol.

Author details

Virgil I. Stenberg[1*] and Ann L. Baldwin[2]

1 University of North Dakota, Bemidji, Minnesota, USA

2 Department of Physiology, University Arizona, Tucson, AZ, USA

*Address all correspondence to: virgilsa@aol.com

References

[1] Burns CM. The history of cortisone discovery and development. Rheumatic Diseases Clinics of North America. 2016;**42**(1):1-14

[2] Hillier SG. Diamonds are forever: The cortisone legacy. The Journal of Endocrinology. 2007;**195**(1):1-6

[3] Sarett LH. A new method for the preparation of 17alpha-hydroxy-20-ketopregnanes. Journal of the American Chemical Society. 1948;**70**:175-185

[4] Sarett LH. The partial synthesis of dehydrocorticosterone acetate. Journal of the American Chemical Society. 1946;**68**:2478-2483

[5] Sarett LH, Arth GE, Lukes RM, Baylor RE, Poos GI, Johns WF, et al. Stereospecific total synthesis of cortisone. Journal of the American Chemical Society. 1952;**74**:4974-4976

[6] Slocumb CH, Polley HF, Ward LE. Diagnosis, treatment and prevention of hypercortisonism in patients with rheumatoid arthritis. Proceedings of the Staff Meetings. Mayo Clinic. 1957;**32**(9):227-238

[7] Rao RT, Scherholz ML, Androulakis IP. Modeling the influence of chronopharmacological administration of synthetic glucocorticoids on the hypothalamic-pituitary-adrenal axis. Chronobiology International. 2018;**12**:1619-1636

[8] Irwin JB, Baldwin AL, Stenberg VI. General theory of inflammation: Patient self-administration of hydrocortisone safely achieves superior control of hydrocortisone-responding disorders by matching dosage with symptom intensity. Journal of Inflammatory Research. 2019;**12**:161-166

[9] Stenberg VI. (mini review) general theory of inflammation. Concise summary of basic principles. Biomedical Journal of Scientific & Technical Research. 2020;**25**(1):18790-18791

[10] Stenberg VI, Bouley MG, Katz BM, Lee KJ, Parmar SS. Negative endocrine control system for inflammation in rats. Agents and Actions. 1990;**29**(3-4):189-195

[11] Stenberg VI, Fiechtner JJ, Rice JR, Miller DR, Johnson LK. Endocrine control of inflammation: Rheumatoid arthritis double-blind, crossover clinical trial. International Journal of Clinical Pharmacology Research. 1992;**12**(1):11-18

[12] Kloppenburg M, Breedveld FC, Terwiel JP, Mallee C, Dijkmans BA. Minocycline in active rheumatoid arthritis. A double-blind, placebo-controlled trial. Arthritis and Rheumatism. 1994;**37**(5):629-636

[13] Panush RS, Stroud RM, Webster EM. Food-induced (allergenic) arthritis. Inflammatory arthritis exacerbated by milk. Arthritis and Rheumatism. 1986;**29**(2):220-226

Chapter 6

Corticosteroids Resistance Diseases Review

Doha Alghamdi and Abdulrahman Alghamdi

Abstract

Glucocorticoids, the main anti-inflammatory medication, are useful for the treatment of many diseases such as inflammation, respiratory diseases, malignancies, etc., but unfortunately, glucocorticoids cannot inhibit inflammation by various mechanisms. The definition of glucocorticoid resistance is loss of efficacy or reduced sensitization over time and increases due to chronic inflammation. It is affecting 30% of glucocorticoid-treated patients. It shows an essential restriction in the treatment of chronic inflammation and malignancies diseases and can be due to the impairment of various mechanisms along the signaling pathway of glucocorticoids. However, glucocorticoids dissociation has been improved to reduce the SE, DIGRAs "receptor of glucocorticoid dissociation agonists" are a group of trial drugs developed to share various wanted as an anti-inflammatory, suppress immunity, or properties of anti-malignancies of traditional steroids medications with lesser adverse events, but it is so hard to dissociate anti-inflammatory effects from adverse effects. Cases with glucocorticoid unresponsive should use other medications with similar mechanisms in inflammation as well as drugs that may change the molecular mechanism of resistance to glucocorticoid. Here, we discuss the evidence that exists for the hypothesis that individual glucocorticoid resistance underlies the problem.

Keywords: glucocorticoid resistance, mechanism of action, diseases, corticosteroids, respiratory diseases

1. Introduction

Glucocorticoid resistance is the absence of the effect of glucocorticoids and the lack of ability of glucocorticoids to produce an effect on the specific tissue. Two ways might be differentiated, generalized unresponsive in which most tissues are (partly) resistant to glucocorticoids, and some specific tissues resistant to glucocorticoids in which just the impacted tissue escapes cortisol action. To date, widespread glucocorticoid resistance has been found in people in some families, in which most cases were asymptomatic despite too much cortisol production [1, 2].

The clinical variability is described by varying levels of glucocorticoid resistance and the differential sensitivity of the mineralocorticoid and the androgen target tissue. A number of criteria for a diagnostic assessment have been well-defined [2], including indices of cortisol excess without the existence of scientific evidence of Cushing's syndrome; resistance to glucocorticoid in numerous tissues such as lymphocytes and the pituitary; and finally, maintenance of hypothalamic–pituitary–adrenal (HPA) axis circadian rhythm and responsiveness to stressors in the existence of cortisol excess.

2. Mechanisms of resistance of glucocorticoid

The genes of pro/anti-inflammation could be stimulated or inhibited by glucocorticoids, as well as having post-transcription. Glucocorticoids hinder the many genes of inflammation that are encouraged in prolong inflammatory diseases, such as bronchial constriction (asthma), via reversing acetylation of histone of stimulated genes of inflammation across binding of ligand glucocorticoid receptors (GR) to costimulatory molecules and recruitment of deacetylase-2 of histone (HDAC2) to the encouraged complex of transcription. In high concentration levels of glucocorticoids – glucocorticoid receptor homodimers interact with locations of gene recognition to encourage transcription within increased acetylation of histone of genes of anti-inflammatory and transcription of several genes associated with GCs SE [3].

However, several chronic inflammatory disease patients (Pt) are unresponsive to glucocorticoid agents such as lung fibrosis caused by bleomycin, chronic pulmonary disease (COPD), and cystic fibrosis raised unresponsive to glucocorticoid is observed in cases with lung diseases. Here are many molecular mechanisms of corticosteroid resistance such as hereditary causes that might establish glucocorticoid responsiveness, a number of abnormalities in work of receptor of glucocorticoid have been explained in fibroblasts from cases with familial glucocorticoid resistance [3].

Numerous SNPs (single nuclear polymorphisms) of glucocorticoid receptors have been associated with the alteration of cellular response to glucocorticoids and a polymorphism of glucocorticoid receptor beta is associated with a reduced response of glucocorticoid trans-repression. These polymorphisms have yet to be linked with resistance to glucocorticoids in inflammatory diseases [3].

There are several methods to modify the receptor of glucocorticoid to diminish their efficacy of nuclear translocation and trans-activation. Phosphorylation may occur because of motivation of p38 mitogen-activated protein kinase (MAPK), which may be encouraged by the cytokine's interleukins such as (IL-2, IL-4, or IL-13), or by MIF (macrophage migration inhibitory factor), of JNK (c-Jun N-terminal kinase) stimulated by pro-inflammatory cytokines or of ERK (extracellular signal-regulated kinase) stimulated by microbial superantigens. In addition, the chronic inflammatory diseases have increased the expression of inducible synthase of NO (iNOS) which produces massive quantities of NO that might encourage glucocorticoid resistance. Also, an increase in the expression of glucocorticoid receptor beta caused by pro-inflammatory cytokines has been observed in glucocorticoid-resistant cases in number of illnesses [3].

In addition, the extreme encouragement of activator protein-1 (AP-1) has been known as a mechanism of glucocorticoid resistance because the activator protein-1 (AP-1) binds glucocorticoid receptor then inhibits its interaction with glucocorticoid receptor element and other transcription factors. Activator protein-1 (AP-1) is a heterodimer of Fos and Jun proteins and might be encouraged by TNF-a (pro-inflammatory cytokines), working within the pathway of c-Jun N-terminal kinase. It describes why the increased inflammation reported in severe inflammatory disease results in secondary glucocorticoid resistance. In elevated c-Jun in de-polymerization of the cytoskeleton, which could also reduce the action of glucocorticoid receptor trans-activating [3].

Cofilin-1 is a depolymerases of actin-binding protein that the cytoskeleton and in gene examinations have been reported as showing increased expression in T-cells from glucocorticoid unresponsive diseases compared to responsive diseases. Thus, the overexpression of cofilin-1 results in glucocorticoid resistance in T-cells [3].

Additionally, one of the most molecular mechanisms of glucocorticoid resistance is abnormal histone acetylation. Acetylation of histone has an essential part in the regulation of inflammatory genes and the mechanism of action of glucocorticoids. Histone deacetylase 2 is significantly decreased in action and expression because of oxidative/nitrative stress so that inflammation becomes resistant to glucocorticoids. The oxygen reactive species also encourages PI3K-delta (phosphoinositide-3-kinase), which causes phosphorylation and deactivation of histone deacetylase 2. So, the oxygen reactive species has an essential mechanism of glucocorticoid resistance and is expanded in most serious and resistance to glucocorticoid diseases [3].

Furthermore, decreased control T cells which cause to decrease in response to glucocorticoid. The interleukine-10 has a role to control the immune cytokine produced by controlling T cells (Treg) in response to glucocorticoids. In decreased glucocorticoid response there is a malfunction of T-helper cells to secrete IL-10 [3].

Also, the inhibitory factor of macrophage migration is a pro-inflammatory cytokine that has strong effects as anti-glucocorticoid and has been associated with various inflammatory diseases. Macrophage migration inhibitory factor has also been involved in glucocorticoid resistance in lung illness [3].

Treatment effects of resistance to glucocorticoid by either selective agonists of the receptor of glucocorticoid (SEGRAs or dissociated steroids) are useful in trans-repression and more effective than trans-activation so have fewer side effects. There are various treatment strategies to control glucocorticoid-unresponsive diseases, but the highly important general methods are to use another anti-inflammatory ("steroid-sparing") medication or to change the mechanisms of action of glucocorticoid resistance (**Figure 1**) [3].

2.1 Corticosteroids resistance due to the interference between the GR and the MAPK signaling pathways

There is a strong interference between the glucocorticoid receptor and mitogen-activated protein kinase (MAPKs) which normally lead to mutual inhibition. In a given inflammatory context, all sensitivity to glucocorticoids is described by multiple interactions of feedback and feedforward between receptors of glucocorticoids and signaling of cytokine-mediated [4, 5]. While various of the actions of anti-inflammatory of glucocorticoids are reached by the receptor of glucocorticoid-mediated inhibition of the activity of mitogen-activated protein kinase, the anti-inflammatory capacity of glucocorticoid is diminished in conditions of extreme activation of mitogen-activated protein kinase (MAPK) [4–6]. Given that chronic MAPK/AP-1-/NF-κB activation is a common denominator in multiple inflammatory diseases, the pharmacological inhibition of a particular MAPK signaling pathway has become an add-on strategy intended to restore the sensitivity of GC [7, 8]. As the interferences between the glucocorticoid receptor and MAPK depend on the affected tissue(s) and are thus disease-dependent, the following sections have been organized according to the distinct pathologies associated with resistance of GC [9].

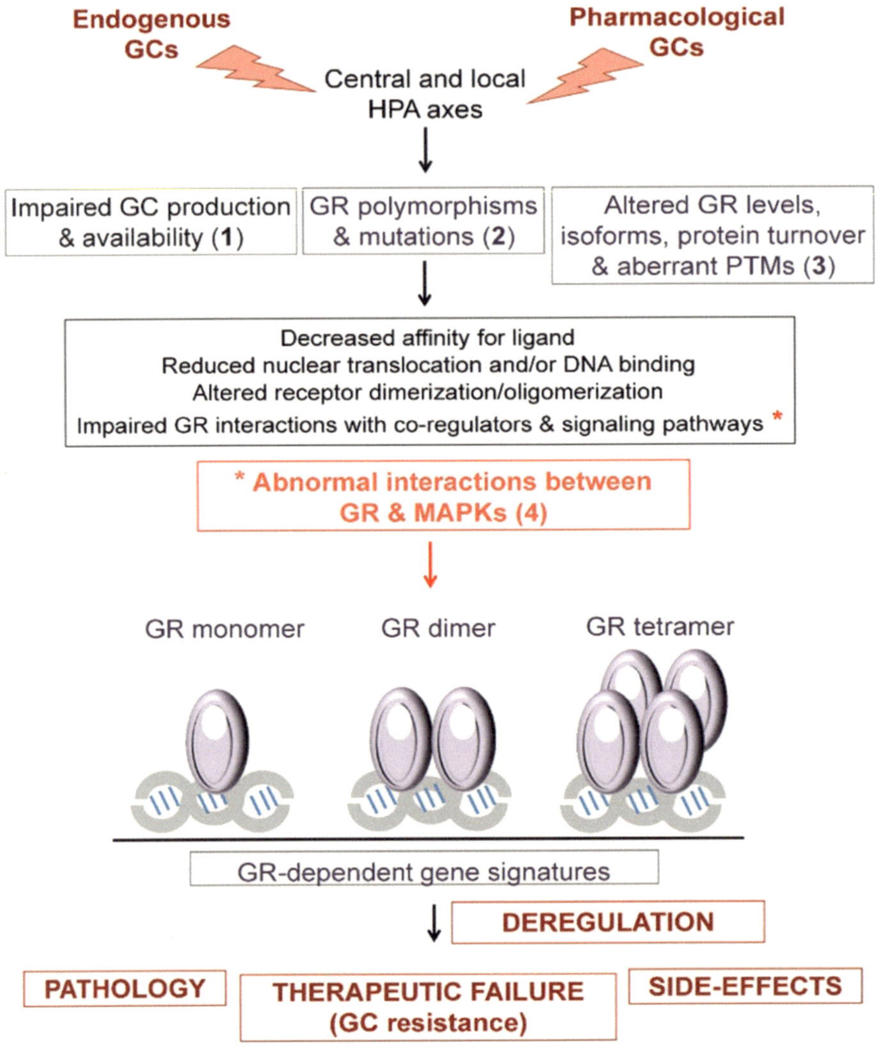

Figure 1.
The mechanisms of glucocorticoid resistance.

3. Respiratory diseases

Respiratory diseases such as asthma, COPD (chronic obstructive pulmonary disease), and pulmonary fibrosis.

3.1 Asthma

Severe cases of asthma are less responsive to corticosteroids than mild cases of asthma, and therefore steroid resistance may be a mechanism contributing to asthma severity. Asthmatic cases who smoke cigarettes also have a reduced response to inhaled corticosteroids (ICSs) and oral corticosteroids, as well as having more severe asthma, a more rapid reduction in the function of the lung with time, and increased cause of death. The acute severe cases of asthma, glucocorticoid resistance relates to elevated levels of pro-inflammatory cytokines with raised expression and the p38 α and β isoforms activity, relative to GC-responsive individuals [10, 11]. The expanded cytokines levels in alveolar macrophages from asthmatic cases with diminished sensitivity to glucocorticoids (GC) lead to stop receptor of glucocorticoid function across its phosphorylation by p38α as well as the reduced induction of DUSP1 by GCs. In chronic pulmonary cases and smoking asthmatics cigarette smoke produces oxygen reactive species (acting through the formation of peroxynitrite) and in acute asthma and COPD intense inflammation generates oxidative stress to impair the activity of HDAC2 histone deacetylase 2. This not only amplifies the inflammatory response to NF-κB activation but also reduces the effect of corticosteroids as anti-inflammatory, as histone deacetylase 2 is now unable to reverse histone acetylation [12].

Subsequent studies revealed that corticosteroids do not inhibit interleukin-2 (IL-2) and interferon-gamma (IFN-g) levels in some cases. Cases with acute bronchial asthma whose clinical manifestations are uncontrolled with maximum amounts of steroid inhalers also display a smaller number of steroids as inhibitory effects on the production of cytokines and chemokines of peripheral monocytes and alveolar macrophages than seen in responsive cases of asthma. In addition, cases with corticosteroid-unresponsive asthma also show decreased skin blanching response to non-systemic corticosteroids, indicating that there may be a generalized abnormality in anti-inflammatory sensitivity to corticosteroids in these cases (**Figure 2**) [12].

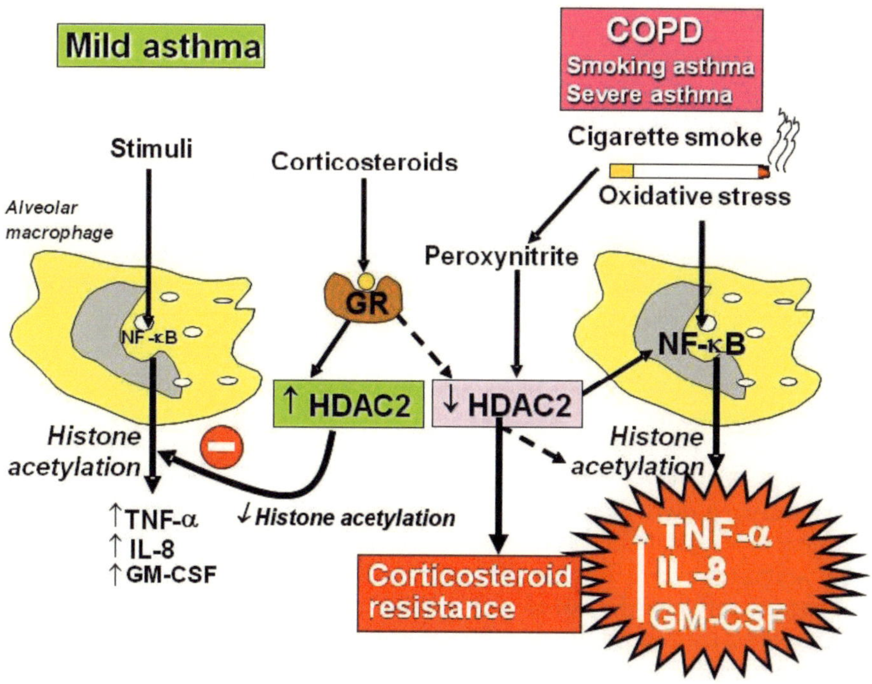

Figure 2.
Corticosteroid resistance in cases of severe asthma and COPD.

3.2 COPD

Chronic obstructive pulmonary disease (COPD) is an inflammatory and irreversible pulmonary disorder that is characterized by inflammation and airway destruction. According to general evidence displayed that there are raised the contents of interleukin-8, MMP-9, phosphoinositide 3-kinase delta, MIF, and glucocorticoids receptor-beta in corticosteroid unresponsive cases than in steroid-responsive cases. In difference, the actions of MAPK phosphatase and histone deacetylase 2 (HDAC2) and mitogen-activated protein kinase phosphatase 1 are attenuated in steroid-resistant cases. Therefore, the inflammation does not significantly contribute to the pathogenesis of the chronic pulmonary disease, but it also produces steroid resistance. Neutrophils, lymphocytes, and macrophages contribute to the cause of steroid resistance [13]. Thus, these cells are potential cell goals for molecular treatment in overcoming steroid resistance. p38α also has a significant role in the pathobiology of chronic pulmonary disease, and its stimulation seems critical for glucocorticoid resistance. While p38 targeting in animal models of chronic pulmonary disease was successful, the outcomes of clinical trials evaluating suppression of p38 for chronic pulmonary disease treatment have been so far disappointing. Presently, the extremely encouraging strategy for the treatment of pulmonary diseases such as bronchial asthma or chronic pulmonary disease depends on the use of inhibition of mitogen-activated protein kinase as add-on therapies to inhaled corticosteroids or BB. A selective p38 inhibitor (GW856553) was described to potentiate inhibition of pro-inflammatory cytokines by glucocorticoids in PBMCs from chronic pulmonary disease cases due to the reduced phosphorylation of glucocorticoid receptor-S211, mediated by p38 [9].

3.3 Pulmonary fibrosis

Nettelbladt and Langenbach reported that there was no effect of MP (methylprednisolone) treatment on bleomycin-caused lung fibrosis in mice models. Also, prednisolone treatment had a partial impact on bleomycin-caused lung fibrosis in animal models [14, 15]. The transforming growth factor-beta is significant to pulmonary inflammation and pulmonary fibrosis. Then corticosteroid treatment administered in the last stages of the disease would likely not hinder the transforming growth factor-beta secretion by alveolar macrophages [16].

The relative resistance to corticosteroid treatment in pulmonary fibrosis seen in several lung diseases patient may be induced by the corticosteroid insensitivity of transforming growth factor-beta secretion by alveolar macrophages. This suggests that the glucocorticoid is effective only in early stages of inflammation [17, 18]. However, at an advanced stage when alveolar macrophages are stimulated to produce the transforming growth factor-beta, thus corticosteroids are useless. Stimulated alveolar macrophages obtained after bleomycin-induced pulmonary injury produced large amounts of the transforming growth factor-beta. Furthermore, the alveolar macrophage secretion of the transforming growth factor-beta is not suppressed by the maximum concentrations of corticosteroids [16]. Hosoya T. and colleagues reported that no effect of corticosteroid in pulmonary inflammation and fibrotic response caused by bleomycin due to of elevated level of IL-4 and was resistant to nonselective glucocorticoid after administration (1 mg/kg/day) in animal model [19]. Also, the interleukin-13-mediated myofibroblast differentiation was not inhibited by corticosteroids [20]. Alghamdi and her colleague found that the corticosteroid has a negative effect on the expression of integrins β3 and β6 in pulmonary fibrosis models and the glucocorticoid has not reduced the edema in lung after 28 days. Also, they found that the corticosteroid was effective in early inflammation but was not effective in advance stage of pulmonary fibrosis based on the histology and immunochemical staining [21].

3.4 Leukemias

Steroids are the most medication used as therapeutic agents for the treatment of all malignancies, such as leukemias, lymphomas, and multiple myeloma, due to their properties of immunosuppressive and anti-inflammatory. Many studies using different cell lines derived from malignancies of human hematology showed that inhibitors of ERK and JNK might restore response to glucocorticoids [22].

The absence-of function mutations, polymorphisms, or downregulation of epigenetics of the gene of NR3C1, glucocorticoids unresponsive in leukemia is commonly caused by changes in other pathways of signal and downstream goals. Indeed, glucocorticoids unresponsive in ALL is consistently linked with changes in the control of programmed cell death, including abnormal expression of Bcl2 family members, deactivation of the tumor suppressor TP53, or overexpression of its suppressor, MDM2. It can also include variations in other transduction signaling pathways including Notch, IL7R/JAK/STAT, phosphatase, and tensin homolog/phosphoinositide 3-kinases/protein kinase b/mammalian target of rapamycin and RAS/mitogen-activated protein kinases. As the apoptotic-related mechanisms of glucocorticoid resistance in immune cells (**Figure 3**) [23].

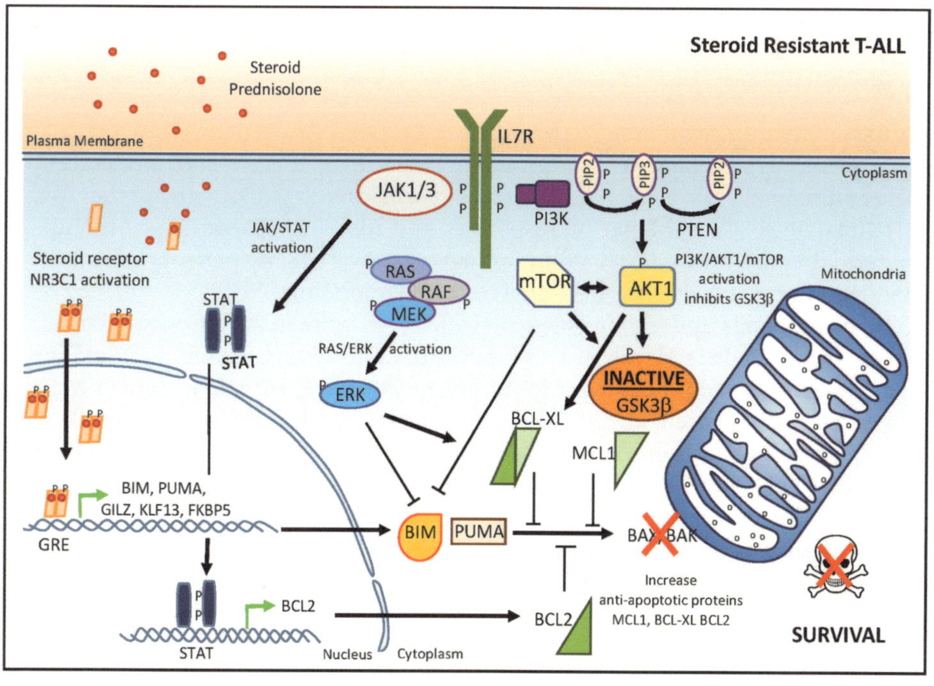

Figure 3.
Molecular mechanisms of glucocorticoid resistance in T-ALL.

4. Autoimmune diseases

Autoimmune diseases such as rheumatoid arthritis and inflammatory bowel diseases (IBD) exhibit diminished efficacy to routine treatments with glucocorticoids.

4.1 Rheumatoid arthritis "RA"

The prevalence of RA is about 0.5–1% of the population, it is a chronic systemic autoimmune disease. The elderly are high risk, in particular females. Among the proteins involved in glucocorticoid resistance, the pro-inflammatory protein MIF, which raises the creation of pro-inflammatory cytokines and positively controls mitogen-activated protein kinase (MAPK) activation, and GILZ, play major roles. The mechanism by which MIF increases mitogen-activated protein kinase (MAPK) phosphorylation involves the suppression of dual specificity protein phosphatase 1 (DUSP1), thus counteracting the effects of anti-inflammatory glucocorticoids [24]. The overexpression of glucocorticoid-induced leucine zipper in endothelial cells decreased adhesion and inflammation by raising the expression of dual specificity protein phosphatase 1 along with suppression of the tumor necrosis factor-induced activation of all mitogen-activated protein kinases [25]. Essentially, MIF-mediated suppression of dual specificity protein phosphatase 1 needs glucocorticoid-induced leucine zipper, exemplifying how feedforward and feedback loops are responsible for modulating the sensitivity to glucocorticoids [24]. These multiple control mechanisms also highlight the significance of the pathway of MAPK/DUSP, as the decrease of dual specificity protein phosphatase 1 (DUSP1) – either due to raised amounts of MIF or deficiency of glucocorticoid-induced leucine zipper (GILZ) – amplifies MAPK-mediated signaling.

4.2 Inflammatory bowel diseases

There are chronic diseases such as Crohn's disease and ulcerative colitis which are linked with uncontrol immune response in mucosa of intestine. Glucocorticoids are prescribed as the major anti-inflammatory treatment in cases with moderate to severe disease. While around half of patients respond to glucocorticoid therapy, approximately 30% exhibit partial responses, and 20% are GC-resistant. Also, upon long-term therapy, around 20% of inflammatory bowel disease patients become dependent, requiring glucocorticoids to continue remission [26].

The mechanisms underlying glucocorticoids resistance in inflammatory bowel diseases include elevated levels of cytokines, such as TNFα, IL-6, and IL-8, and low IL-10, in steroid-resistant comparative to steroid sensitive, with activation of the mitogen-activated protein kinase (MAPK) /AP-1 and nuclear factor κB (NF-κB) pathways. Macrophage inhibitory factor (MIF) is also implicated in the pathogenesis of ulcerative colitis through activation of cytokines and subsequent effects of anti-steroid [27]. As most cytokines are goals of main pro-inflammatory linked TFs, this scenario constitutes an auto-amplification loop for glucocorticoids resistance.

5. Conclusion

Many diseases are resistant to corticosteroids with explanation of resistance but mainly molecular mechanism of this resistance is the activation of the mitogen-activated protein kinases (MAPKs) and/or alterations in expression of their regulators, the dual-specific phosphatases (DUSPs), transforming growth factor-beta.

Acknowledgements

First, thanks to Allah for the blessings and help. Then, I would like to thank all those people who shared me their knowledge and experiences and supported me.

I wish to thank my committee members who were more than generous with their expertise and precious time.

A special feeling of gratitude to my parents, my husband, my daughter, my sister, and my brothers who encouraged me and pushed me to do my best.

My parents and my husband have never left my side and always support me.

Conflict of interest

The authors declare no conflict of interest.

Author details

Doha Alghamdi[1,2]* and Abdulrahman Alghamdi[3]

1 Pharmacology Department, Faculty of Medicine, King Abdulaziz University, Jeddah, Saudi Arabia

2 Pharmacology Department, King Abdulaziz University, Jeddah, Saudi Arabia

3 Community Pharmacy, Jeddah, Saudi Arabia

*Address all correspondence to: dohaalghamdi93@gmail.com

References

[1] Lamberts S et al. Clinical aspects of glucocorticoid sensitivity. Steroids. 1996;**61**(4):157-160

[2] Chrousos GP, Detera-Wadleigh SD, Karl M. Syndromes of glucocorticoid resistance. Annals of Internal Medicine. 1993;**119**(11):1113-1124

[3] Barnes PJ. Mechanisms and resistance in glucocorticoid control of inflammation. The Journal of Steroid Biochemistry and Molecular Biology. 2010;**120**(2-3):76-85

[4] Rodriguez JM et al. Glucocorticoid resistance in chronic diseases. Steroids. 2016;**115**:182-192

[5] Newton R et al. Glucocorticoid and cytokine crosstalk: Feedback, feedforward, and co-regulatory interactions determine repression or resistance. Journal of Biological Chemistry. 2017;**292**(17):7163-7172

[6] Beck IM et al. Crosstalk in inflammation: The interplay of glucocorticoid receptor-based mechanisms and kinases and phosphatases. Endocrine Reviews. 2009;**30**(7):830-882

[7] Cain DW, Cidlowski JA. Specificity and sensitivity of glucocorticoid signaling in health and disease. Best Practice & Research Clinical Endocrinology & Metabolism. 2015;**29**(4):545-556

[8] De Bosscher K et al. Nuclear receptor crosstalk—Defining the mechanisms for therapeutic innovation. Nature Reviews Endocrinology. 2020;**16**(7):363-377

[9] Sevilla LM et al. Glucocorticoid resistance: Interference between the glucocorticoid receptor and the MAPK Signalling pathways. International Journal of Molecular Sciences. 2021;**22**(18):10049

[10] Quax RA et al. Glucocorticoid sensitivity in health and disease. Nature Reviews Endocrinology. 2013;**9**(11):670-686

[11] Petta I et al. The interactome of the glucocorticoid receptor and its influence on the actions of glucocorticoids in combatting inflammatory and infectious diseases. Microbiology and Molecular Biology Reviews. 2016;**80**(2):495-522

[12] Barnes PJ. Corticosteroid resistance in patients with asthma and chronic obstructive pulmonary disease. Journal of Allergy and Clinical Immunology. 2013;**131**(3):636-645

[13] Jiang Z, Zhu L. Update on molecular mechanisms of corticosteroid resistance in chronic obstructive pulmonary disease. Pulmonary Pharmacology & Therapeutics. 2016;**37**:1-8

[14] Nettelbladt O, Tengblad A, Hallgren R. High-dose corticosteroids during bleomycin-induced alveolitis in the rat do not suppress the accumulation of hyaluronan (hyaluronic acid) in lung tissue. European Respiratory Journal. 1990;**3**(4):421-428

[15] Langenbach SY et al. Resistance of fibrogenic responses to glucocorticoid and 2-methoxyestradiol in bleomycin-induced lung fibrosis in mice. Canadian Journal of Physiology and Pharmacology. 2007;**85**(7):727-738

[16] Khalil N et al. Regulation of alveolar macrophage transforming growth factor-beta secretion by

corticosteroids in bleomycin-induced pulmonary inflammation in the rat. The Journal of Clinical Investigation. 1993;**92**(4):1812-1818

[17] Izbicki G et al. Time course of bleomycin-induced lung fibrosis. International Journal of Experimental Pathology. 2002;**83**(3):111-119

[18] Matsuyama H et al. Acute lung inflammation and ventilator-induced lung injury caused by ATP via the P2Y receptors: An experimental study. Respiratory Research. 2008;**9**(1):1-13

[19] Hosoya T. Steroid resistance and lung-tissue cytokines in experimental bleomycin-induced lung fibrosis. The Japanese Journal of Thoracic Diseases. 1997;**35**(7):766-775

[20] Wilson M, Wynn T. Pulmonary fibrosis: Pathogenesis, etiology and regulation. Mucosal Immunology. 2009;**2**(2):103-121

[21] Alghamdi DO, Kawy HSA, Damanhouri ZA. Nintedanib reduces corticosteroid resistance pulmonary fibrosis induced by bleomycin in mice by increasing the expression of β3 & β6 integrins. Research Square. 2021

[22] Olivas-Aguirre M et al. Overcoming glucocorticoid resistance in acute lymphoblastic leukemia: Repurposed drugs can improve the protocol. Frontiers in Oncology. 2021;**11**:617937

[23] Garza AS et al. Converting cell lines representing hematological malignancies from glucocorticoid-resistant to glucocorticoid-sensitive: Signaling pathway interactions. Leukemia Research. 2009;**33**(5):717-727

[24] Fan H et al. Macrophage migration inhibitory factor inhibits the Antiinflammatory effects of glucocorticoids via glucocorticoid-induced leucine zipper. Arthritis & Rheumatology. 2014;**66**(8):2059-2070

[25] Cheng Q et al. GILZ overexpression inhibits endothelial cell adhesive function through regulation of NF-κB and MAPK activity. The Journal of Immunology. 2013;**191**(1):424-433

[26] Dubois-Camacho K et al. Glucocorticosteroid therapy in inflammatory bowel diseases: From clinical practice to molecular biology. World Journal of Gastroenterology. 2017;**23**(36):6628

[27] De Iudicibus S et al. Molecular mechanism of glucocorticoid resistance in inflammatory bowel disease. World Journal of Gastroenterology: WJG. 2011;**17**(9):1095

Chapter 7

Prevalence and Predictive Factors of Low-Bone Mineral Density in Patients with Addison Disease on Long-Term Corticosteroid Replacement Therapy

Dhouha Ben Salah and Khouloud Boujelben

Abstract

Addison disease (AD) is associated with high risk of decreased bone mineral density (BMD) and osteoporosis. Causes are complex, including lifelong glucocorticoid replacement therapy. The aim of our study was to assess the influence of glucorticoid replacement therapy on BMD among patients with AD and determine predictive factors of low BMD. A descriptive and analytical cross-sectional study was conducted at the department of endocrinology-diabetology at HediChaker Hospital, including 50 patients with AD for at least 5 years. Serum levels of bone turnover markers were measured and BMD was determined. The mean age of patients was 49.5 ± 13.9 years. Received average daily dose of hydrocortisone (HC) was 27.4 ± 6.7 mg. Mean cumulative HC dose was 374.636 ± 283.821 mg. Mean T-score at lumbar spine and femoral neck was –0.61 ± 1.06 (range,–4.2–1.1) and –1.18 ± 1.33 (range,–2.9–1.3), respectively. Low BMD was observed in 48% of patients. No fracture was observed. Patients who developed osteoporosis were significantly older than those with normal BMD ($p = 0.018$). Menopause was a significant predictor of incident osteoporosis ($p = 0.006$). Furthermore, osteoporosis was significantly more prevalent among females ($p = 0.046$). Daily and cumulative HC dose were higher in patients with osteoporosis than those with normal osteodensitometry. Glucocorticoid replacement therapy in AD may induce bone loss. Thus, glucocorticoid therapy must be adjusted to the lowest tolerable dose.

Keywords: Addison disease, glucocorticoid replacement therapy, bone mineral density, osteoporosis, bone health

1. Introduction

Patients with AD lack sufficient endogenous secretion of glucocorticoids [1]. The treatment of AD usually involves lifelong glucocorticoid replacement therapy, most usually oral hydrocortisone (HC). Nevertheless, glucocorticoid replacement therapy usually produces cortisol levels higher than the normal physiological endogenous secretion [2].

In spite of the fact that prolonged substitution with glucocorticoids carries a significant risk of bone loss by a proapoptotic action on osteoblasts, promoting osteoclastic activity [3], and decreasing intestinal calcium absorption [4], BMD assessment is not indicated in regular follow-up of patients with PAI. To date, few researches have focused on skeletal health in patients with AD. The majority of studies included relatively small series of patients and reported variable results between BMD, glucocorticoid dose, duration disease (duration therapy), glucocorticoid regimens, and cumulative dose [5–9]. Several studies reported normal BMD [8], while others showed reduced density in all or some bone sites [6]. Thus, the aim of our study was to assess the impact of glucocorticoid replacement therapy on bone density in patients with AD and determine predictive factors of low BMD in this population.

2. Materials and methods

2.1 Study design, area, and period

A cross-sectional study was carried out at the department of Endocrinology-Diabetology of Hedi Chaker Academic Hospital -Sfax –Tunisia, from March 2020 to July 2021. In addition, the study comprised retrospective collection of clinical data from patients' medical records.

Inclusion criteria were patients with AD and disease duration of at least 5 years.

Patients under the age of 18 years, presenting conditions that may affect bone homeostasis (hypogonadism except physiological menopause, primary hyperparathyroidism, hyperthyroidism, rheumatoid arthritis, chronic renal failure, hepatocellular dysfunction, hemochromatosis, chronic pancreatitis, gastrointestinal diseases that cause malabsorption syndrome and prolonged immobilization), taking drugs that may interfere with bone metabolism (heparin, vitamin K antagonist, thiazide diuretics, calcitonin, bisphosphonates, anticonvulsant drugs and hormone therapy for menopause) were excluded.

Patients meeting the inclusion criteria were recruited. All patients gave their written informed consent before being assessed.

A total of 80 patients with AD were contacted, 37.5% of the patients did not respond or declined to be assessed. Lastly, 50 patients with AD were recruited in the present study.

The data of patients including age, gender, age at diagnosis, disease duration, physical activity, Body Mass Index (BMI), and menopausal status for female patients were assessed.

2.2 Glucocorticoid treatment

All patients were treated with HC.

The average daily HC doses were assessed (mg and mg/kg) and were adjusted for body surface area (mg/m^2).

As well, cumulative glucocorticoid dose, defined as the cumulative amount of glucocorticoid intake since the time of diagnosis to the date of BMD measurement, was estimated by summing partial cumulative doses for each time period during which the dose remained constant.

To determine partial cumulative dose, we have used the following formula:

$$\left[\text{daily hydrocortisone dose (in milligrams or in milligrams/kg) x time period}\right].$$

2.3 Biochemical markers of bone turnover

Serum samples of patients were collected to measure calcium, phosphorus, alkaline phosphatase (ALP), vitamin D, and parathyroid hormone (PTH)).

An ALP level above 150 IU/l was considered as high.

PTH (normal range, 15–65 pg./ml) and vitamin D (normal range, 30–100 ng/ml) were measured by electrochemiluminescence immunoassay (ECLIA).

2.4 BMD

BMD was evaluated using dual-energy X-ray absorptiometry (DEXA), at the lumbar spine (L1–L4) (trabecular bone) and femoral neck (cortical bone) sites, based on a standard protocol.

The results were expressed as BMD in g/cm^2, T- and Z- scores expressed as standard deviation (SD), in both lumbar and femoral sites.

Referring to the World Health Organization (WHO) classification, osteoporosis is defined as a T-score ≤ 2.5 SD and osteopenia as a T-score between -2.5 and -1 SD [10].

2.5 Statistical analysis

Statistical analysis of data was done by using the "Statistical Package for Social Sciences" (SPSS) version 25.

Thus, we performed a univariate analysis based on the comparison of means on paired series using the Student test and the non-parametric Mann–Whitney–Wilcoxon test for unpaired series.

Several regression analyses were achieved to recognize factors impacting BMD in patients with AD. Current BMD was correlated with cumulative and average daily glucocorticoid doses, as well as with clinical and laboratory data.

A point estimate of Odds ratio (OR) with a 95% confidence interval was determined to evaluate the strength of relationship.

Statistical significance was accepted if p-value <0.05.

3. Results

3.1 Clinical descriptive data

Median age of patients was 49.5 ± 13.9 years old with extremes ranging from 18 to 78 years. There were 40 females and 10 males.

The majority of patients (70%) were aged between 40 and 50 years old. Ten percent of patients were smokers.

Two thirds (66%) of patients were not physically active.

Approximately 42.5% of females were postmenopausal. All patients took neither calcium oral supplementation nor estrogen replacement therapy.

Average age at diagnosis of AD was 35.5 ± 14.6 years (range, 0–70 years).

Average AD duration was 13.9 ± 8.7 years (range, 5–35 years).

Patients' average weight was 72.5 kg (range, 62–107 kg), and average BMI was estimated at 28.1 kg/m^2 (range, 21.2–45.8 kg/m^2).

Overweight was noted in 48% of patients and obesity in 26%.

3.2 Glucocorticoid treatment

Average daily HC dose at the time of AD diagnosis was 25.7 ± 9.1 mg (range, 15–50 mg) corresponding to 0.47 ± 0.21 mg/kg (range, 8–1.08 mg/kg) and an average daily dose adjusted for body surface area of 16.29 ± 7.54 mg/m^2 (range, 15.6–37.94 mg/m^2).

HC was prescribed twice a day for 67% of patients with an initial daily dose greater than 30 mg in 44% of patients.

During follow-up, the average daily HC dose was 27.4 ± 6.7 mg (range, 15–42.1 mg) corresponding to 0.388 ± 0.128 mg/kg (range, 0.175–0.711 mg/kg) and a mean dose per body surface area of 14.836 ± 4.658 mg/m^2 (7.486–31.460 mg/m^2) (**Figure 1**).

Thirty-nine (78%) patients received a mean daily HC dose greater than 11 mg/m^2.

Cumulative HC dose was 374.636 ± 283.821 mg (range, 60–1184, 94 mg) corresponding to 5.924 ± 4.648 mg/kg (range, 0.875–17.238 mg/kg).

3.3 Bone turnover markers

Mean serum calcium and phosphorus levels were 2.29 ± 0.13 mmol/l (range, 1.9–2.55 mmol/l) and 1.10 ± 0.18 mmol/l (range, 0.8–1.66 mmol/l), respectively.

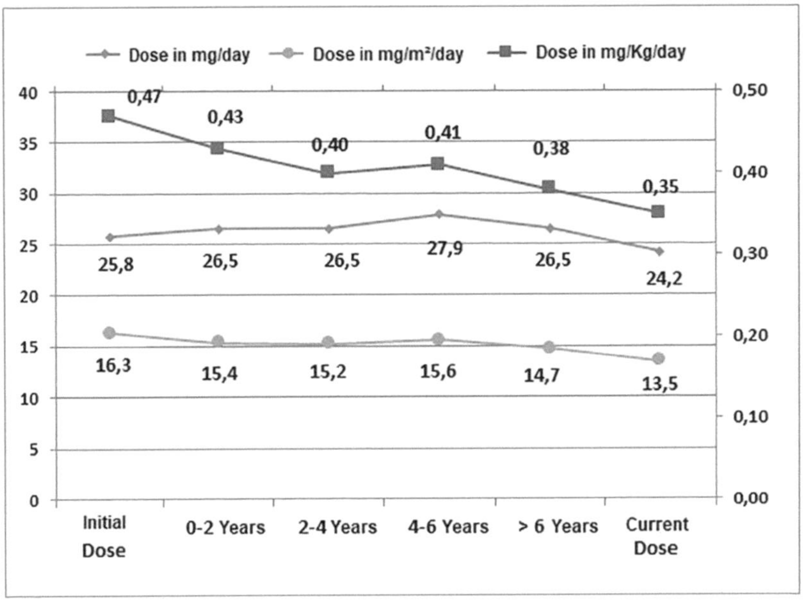

Figure 1.
Average daily HC dose during follow up of patients with AD.

Hypocalcemia was observed in 18% of patients after a mean AD duration of 11.9 ± 7.1 years (range, 4–26 years) and a mean cumulative HC dose of 317.7 ± 211.7 mg (range, 75–702 mg).

In fact, hypocalcemia had no significant correlation with none of glucocorticoid replacement duration (p = 0.397) or glucocorticoid dose (p = 0.680).

Mean ALP was 77.2 ± 28.5 IU/l (range, 15–190 IU/l). Patients presenting an increased ALP level (18%) received higher cumulative HC intake but without statistical significance (413.4 ± 348 mg versus 365.5 ± 271 mg, p = 0.7).

Mean vitamin D level was 22.28 ± 14.14 ng/ml (range, 5.6–78.6 ng/ml). Hypovitaminosis D was observed in 66% of patients.

All patients with hypocalcemia had hypovitaminosis D.

Mean PTH level was 51.79 ± 23.84 pg./ml (range, 16.36–139 pg./ml). An elevated PTH level was observed in 20% of patients who presented with all vitamin D deficiency.

Finally, biochemical parameters of bone turnover in patients with AD showed no significant correlation with none of AD duration or glucocorticoid dose.

3.4 BMD in patients with AD

The average BMD at lumbar spine and femoral neck was 0.928 ± 0.174 g/cm^2 (range, 0.596–1287 g/cm^2) and 0.945 ± 0.145 g/cm^2, (range, 0.687–1.265 g/cm^2), respectively.

The data on BMD at both lumbar spine and femoral neck are shown in **Table 1**.

The T-scores at lumbar spine were lower than at femoral neck. Similarly, lumbar spine Z-scores were lower than at femoral site.

Twenty-four (48%) patients had reduced BMD (less than 2 standard deviations [SD] of the mean value of an age-matched reference population). Among these patients, 12 had osteoporosis, corresponding to 24% of all patients including in our study. Also, osteopenia was observed in 24% of patients.

But, none had a history of spontaneous or traumatic fracture.

3.5 Predictive factors for low BMD in patients with AD

Patients with low BMD were significantly older than those with normal BMD (53.6 ± 11.8 years versus 45.17 ± 15.04 years, p = 0.04).

As well, BMD was significantly more frequent in postmenopausal women (risk ratio = 3.7, p = 0.049) (p = 0.049).

No significant BMD variation was observed according to BMI (p = 0.71) or AD duration (p = 0.79).

PTH level was higher in patients with decreased BMD but without a statistically significant association (56 ± 21.8 pg./ml versus 48.1 ± 25.4 pg./ml, p = 0.1).

Scores (SD)	Mean ± SD	Minimum–Maximum
T-score lumbar spine (L1–L4)	-1.18 ± 1.33	4.2-1.1
T-score femoral neck	−0.61 ± 1.06	−2.9-1.3
Z-score lumbar spine (L1–L4)	−0.92 ± 1.18	3.5-1.3
Z-score femoral neck	−0.28 ± 0.79	−1.8-1.3

Abbreviation: SD, standard deviation.

Table 1.
Results of bone densitometry in lumbar spine and femoral neck.

Also, vitamin D level was lower in patients presenting low BMD compared to those with normal BMD but still without statistically significant correlation (19 ± 10.2 ng/ml versus 25.2 ± 16.6 ng/ml, p = 0.2).

As for glucocorticoid therapy dose, although it was higher in patients with reduced BMD, no correlation was observed between cumulative HC dose and low BMD.

Table 2 shows daily and cumulative glucocorticoid dose variation between patients with normal BMD and those with low bone mass.

3.6 Predictive factors for osteoporosis in patients with AD

Patients who developed osteoporosis were significantly older than those with normal BMD (p = 0.018). The menopause was also a significant predictor of incident osteoporosis (p = 0.006). Furthermore, osteoporosis was significantly more prevalent

Glucocorticoid dose	Normal BMD (n = 30)	Low BMD (n = 20)	p-value
Daily dose (mg)	25.6 ± 6.3	26.0 ± 7.3	0.969
Daily dose (mg/kg)	0.4 ± 0.1	0.4 ± 0.1	0.336
Daily dose per body surface (mg/m^2)	15.0 ± 4.8	14.7 ± 4.6	0.892
Cumulative dose (mg)	338.9 ± 236.8	408.9 ± 324	0.774
Cumulative dose (mg/kg)	5.0 ± 3.9	6.8 ± 5.2	0.322

Abbreviation: BMD, bone mineral density.

Table 2.
Correlation between glucocorticoid dose and BMD.

Clinical/Laboratory data		No osteoporosis (n = 30)	Osteoporosis (n = 12)	p-value
Age (year)		46.7 ± 13.6	58.4 ± 11.4	0.018
Gender	Male	10 (20%)	0 (0%)	0.046
	Female	28 (56%)	12 (24%)	
Menopause		8 (21%)	9 (75%)	0.006
BMI (kg/m^2)	Normal BMI [5–25]	23 (54.8%)	7 (16.7%)	0.514
	Overweight [25–30]	7 (16.7%)	1 (2.4%)	
	Obesity (>30)	2 (4.8%)	2 (4.8%)	
Disease duration		13.2 ± 8.0	16.4 ± 10.9	0.412
Parathyroid hormone (pg/ml)		50.6 ± 23.9	55.8 ± 24.3	0.375
Vitamin D (ng/ml)		23.7 ± 14.9	17.3 ± 9.9	0.175
Calcemia (mmol/I)		2.3 ± 0.1	2.3 ± 0.1	0.510
Phosphoremia (mmol/l)		1.1 ± 0.2	1.2 ± 0.2	0.122
Alcaline phosphatase (IU/I)		72.3 ± 20.3	92.9 ± 43.2	0.275

Abbreviation: BMI, body mass index.

Table 3.
Relationships between osteoporosis and patients' clinical/laboratory data.

Glucocorticoid dose	No osteoporosis (n = 30)	Osteoporosis (n = 12)	p-value
Daily dose (mg)	25.6 ± 6.3	26.5 ± 8.3	0.954
Daily dose (mg/kg)	0.4 ± 0.1	0.4 ± 0.2	0.146
Daily dose per body surface (mg/m^2)	14.7 ± 4.6	15.3 ± 5.0	0.683
Cumulative dose (mg)	344.6 ± 245.5	462.2 ± 373.2	0.487
Cumulative dose (mg/kg)	5.5 ± 4.3	7.0 ± 5.6	0.407

Table 4.
Correlation between glucocorticoid dose and BMD.

among females (p = 0.046). No significant association was found between osteoporosis and AD duration as shown in **Table 3**.

Then, we studied the effect of glucocorticoid replacement therapy on BMD and the occurrence of osteoporosis in patients with AD.

Daily and cumulative HC doses were higher in patients with osteoporosis than those with normal osteodensitometry (26.5 ± 8.3 mg/day versus 25.6 ± 6.3 mg/day; 462.2 ± 373.2 mg versus 344.6 ± 245.5 mg), but none of these factors had a significant impact on the occurrence of osteoporosis as shown in **Table 4**.

4. Discussion

4.1 Glucocorticoid effects on calcium-phosphorus metabolism and bone health

Glucocorticoid therapy is the primary cause of secondary osteoporosis.

This complication is essentially dependent on the dose and duration of glucocorticoid treatment [12].

According to the medical literature, bone loss occurs in two stages: an early stage characterized by a sharp decline in BMD of between 6 and 12% over the first year of treatment, followed by a long-term phase where BMD slowly declines at a rate of roughly 3% per year [12, 13].

Thus, early in the course of treatment, osteoporotic fractures are significantly more common as a result of high-dose synthetic corticosteroid therapy [14, 15].

The bone effects of glucocorticoid are complex, resulting from direct effects on bone tissue and indirect repercussions on calcium homeostasis and sex steroid production.

Glucocorticoids exert a proapoptotic effect on osteoblasts and osteocytes [16]. Type I collagen, a vital component of bone, cannot be synthesized.

The main impact of glucocorticoids on bone cell function is the reduction of osteoformation activity by osteoblasts, resulting in a low osteocalcin level [16].

Glucocorticoids also promote bone resorption through other various mechanisms, such as raising RANKL (Receptor Activator of Nuclear Factor κB Ligand) synthesis and reducing in osteoprotegerin level, an osteoclastogenesis inhibitor.

In addition, glucocorticoids affect phosphocalcic metabolism by decreasing intestinal calcium absorption by inhibiting its transport and increasing renal calcium excretion [4, 17]. This leads to hypocalcemia and consequently secondary hyperparathyroidism [11, 18].

Finally, glucocorticoids influence gonadal hormone production by inducing hypogonadism and may in some situations also reduce adrenal androgens production [16].

In fact, sex steroids promote osteoblast proliferation and maturation, while they inhibit osteoclastic activity conversely, which results in an optimal concentration of calcium at sites of bone mineralization. Estrogens also act directly on bone tissue where their main effect is to inhibit osteoclastic activity [19].

As prescribed at supraphysiological levels, glucocorticoid replacement therapy in AD could have similar effects on phosphocalcic metabolism and the same induced bone side repercussions [20, 21].

4.2 Bone turnover markers in patients with AD

In our study, 18% of the patients had hypocalcemia after a mean disease duration of 11.9 ± 7.1 years, without statistically significant association with HC dose or disease duration.

Our findings are in agreement with those of Suliman et al. [22] reporting low levels of ionized calcium in patients with AD compared to controls ($p < 0.001$) but without a significant association with HC dose.

Indeed, hypocalcemia is uncommon in isolated AD. The majority of reported cases of hypocalcemia were part of an autoimmune polyendocrinopathy (AIP) associating AD with celiac disease or hypoparathyroidism [23, 24].

In our study, the vitamin D deficiency observed in 66% of patients could partly explain this hypocalcemia.

Some data in medical literature suggested an association between vitamin D deficiency and AD. Ramagopalan et al. [25] observed a significantly high prevalence of autoimmune diseases including AD among 13,260 patients hospitalized for hypovitaminosis D in a British center. It was proposed that vitamin D deficiency may disrupt the immune response and induce inflammatory responses that would trigger the development of autoimmune diseases.

In addition, it has recently been demonstrated that skin hyperpigmentation reduces the skin's capacity to generate vitamin D3 when ultraviolet B radiation is present [26].

The high melanin content of their skin may account for hypovitaminosis D, which often observed in patients with AD.

4.3 BMD in patients with AD

Several researches have been interested in assessing BMD in AD.

In our series, low BMD was observed in almost half of the patients (48%) of whom 24% had femoral and/or vertebral osteoporosis.

The mean lumbar spine and femoral neck Z-scores were low (−0.92 ± 1.18 and − 0.28 DS, respectively) but remained within the normal range (between −2 and + 2).

Despite the fact that their findings are conflicting, the majority of studies revealed that patients with AD experience a more frequent decline in BMD than the general population [27–30].

Zelissen et al. [6] were the first to find in 1994 the bone loss in 91 patients with AD, with an estimated prevalence of 32% in women and 7% in men.

According to Leelarathna et al. [28], more than 50% of AD patients included in their study (n = 292) had osteopenia, and one patient out of 5 developed osteoporosis. Bone demineralization was predominant in the lumbar spine, in agreement with our results.

Other studies did not observe a significant decrease in BMD in patients with AD [8, 31].

Camozzi et al. [32] analyzed BMD in 87 patients with AD compared to 81 healthy controls, and no higher risk of reduced BMD was found in AD patients in comparison with controls.

Table 5 summarizes the results of several studies that have analyzed BMD in patients with AD.

Some studies have also investigated the risk of osteoporotic fractures in AD patients.

Study, reference number	Year	Country	Population	Study design	Results
Zellissen [6]	1994	Netherlands	91 AD	Cross-sectional	Decreased BMD in 32% of women and 7% of men.
Florkowski [33]	1994	New Zealand	14 AD	Observational	Women with AD showed a higher risk of low BMD in comparison with males.
Braatvedt [30]	1999	New Zealand	29 AD	Observational	A significant decrease in BMD in males
Heureux [27]	2000	France	24 AD	Prospective	More than half of patients (58%) had osteoporosis.
Jódar [31]	2003	Spain	25 AD	Cross-sectional	No significant reduction of BMD in patients with AD.
Arlt [24]	2006	United Kingdom	23 AD 23 CI	Cross-sectional	BMD in patients with AD is generally normal and does not require long-term monitoring.
Levås [29]	2009	Norway United Kingdom New Zealand	292 AD	Cross-sectional	Z-score was significantly reduced at both femoral neck (−0.28 SD in Norway and − 0.21 SD in New Zealand) and lumbar spine (−0.17 SD in Norway and − 0.57 SD in New Zealand).
Leelarathna [28]	2010	United Kingdom	48 AD	Retrospective	More than half of patients with AD had osteopenia and 1 in 5 patients had osteoporosis.
Chandy [34]	2016	India	41 AD	Cross-sectional	Osteoporosis was observed in 43% of patients with AD versus 25% in control patients.
Camozzi [32]	2018	Italy	87 AD	Cross-sectional	No significant difference in BMD was observed between patients with AD and healthy controls.
Our study	2021	Tunisia	50 AD	Cross-sectional	Low BMD was observed in 48% of patients, 24% of whom had osteoporosis.

Abbreviation: AD, Addison Disease; CI, Corticotropic Insufficiency; BMD, Bone Mineral Density.

Table 5.
Synopsis of main clinical studies analyzing BMD in patients with AD.

A Swedish study examined the risk of hip fracture in patients with AD who showed a higher risk compared to healthy controls (6.9 vs. 2.7% in controls; $p < 0.001$) [35].

Similarly, Camozzi et al. [32] showed that 31.1% of patients with AD had at least one vertebral fracture related to osteoporosis, compared with only 12.8% of control subjects (odds ratio = 3.09).

4.4 Predictive factors of low BMD in patients with AD

***Disease duration**

Lee et al. [36] have demonstrated that bone loss occurs early in AD, even before diagnosis, since glucocorticoids promote osteoblastic precursor differentiation, and therefore, hypocorticism might result in osteoblastic immaturity and reduced bone mass.

Studies investigating the correlation between the age of AD and bone status are heterogeneous, and their results are contradictory. However, the majority of findings have not reported a correlation between disease duration and BMD in patients with AD [6, 8, 28, 31, 34].

***Age**

Bone demineralization in the general population begins progressively from the age of 25 years and increases linearly with age.

In fact, aging leads to an osteoformation decrease by a reduction of osteoblast activity as well as an acceleration of bone resorption due to a state of hyperparathyroidism secondary to the hypovitaminosis D frequently observed in the elderly subject.

This bone loss increases rapidly after menopause in women and remains constant in men [37, 38].

In AD patients, the curve of bone mass evolution according to age is similar to that of the general population.

Thus, Jodar et al. [31] observed that no BMD variation according to age was found. Similarly, Valero et al. [39] in their cross-sectional study of 30 AD patients with an average age of 52.2 years reported the same result.

In our study, patients with low BMD were older than those with normal BMD but without significant differences.

***Menopause**

Various studies studying BMD in AD patients reported a more frequent bone loss (osteopenia and/or osteoporosis) in menopausal women [5, 32, 33, 39].

In a comparative study reported by Camozzi et al. [32], none of the menopausal women in the control group experienced an osteoporotic fracture, while menopausal AD women had a fracture rate of 53%.

This finding suggests a major impact of glucocorticoid replacement therapy in the occurrence of atraumatic fractures in menopausal AD women.

***Glucocorticoid dose**

Most of studies concur that optimal glucocorticoid replacement therapy requires a daily dose of 15 to 20 mg equivalent to 10–12 mg/m^2 [1, 40].

A recent Endocrine Society Clinical Practice Guideline recommended a daily HC dose of 15–25 mg for patients with AD [2]. But most of AD patients seemed to be on supraphysiological glucocorticoid doses, resulting in catabolic repercussions on bone health.

In our study, 78% of patients received a daily HC dose greater than 11 mg/m^2. Higher mean cumulative HC doses, particularly in patients with osteoporosis, were observed in patients with low BMD.

Several studies have examined the impact of HC dose on bone health in patients with AD [5, 6, 30, 41].

In a study involving 91 patients with AD, Zelissen et al. [6] observed that mean BMD was negatively correlated with current glucocorticoid dose but only in men ($p = 0.032$). Patients treated with a daily HC dose of less than 13.6 mg/m^2 had normal BMD instead of those receiving more than 16.4 mg/m^2.

In another prospective study, Schulz et al. [5] reported that HC dose reduction from 30.8 ± 8.5 mg/d to 21.4 ± 7.2 mg/d induced a significant improvement in lumbar spine and femoral Z-scores in 90 AD patients (from -0.93 ± 1.2 to -0.65 ± 1.5 ($p < 0.05$) and from -0.40 ± 1.0 to -0.28 ± 1.0 ($p < 0.05$), respectively) [5].

In contrast, Koetz et al. observed that lower glucocorticoid dose did not improve BMD in 81 AD patients [8] .

These same findings were also reported by Jodar et al. [31], Florkowski et al. [33], Valero et al. [39], and Chandy et al. studies [34].

Finally, the vast majority of medical researches concur that high cumulative glucocorticoid dose is associated with an increased prevalence of bone demineralization in AD patients.

Table 6 summarizes several studies assessing glucocorticoid dose's impact on BMD in patients with AD.

Study, reference number	Year	Country	Population	Study design	HC dose	Impact of glucocorticoid dose on BMD
Zellissen [6]	1994	Netherlands	91 AD	Cross-sectional	29.2 ± 7.0 mg/day	Significant correlation between daily HC dose and low BMD ($p = 0.032$) in men.
Valero [39]	1994	Spain	25 AD	Cross-sectional	30 mg/day	No correlation was found
Florkowski [33]	1994	New-Zealand	14 AD	Cross-sectional	27.6 ± 6.1 mg/day	No correlation was found
Braatvedt [30]	1999	New Zealand	29 AD	Observational	24 + 2.4 mg/day CD:2.28 + 0.64 g/kg	Negative correlation between daily and cumulative glucocorticoid dose and BMD
Jódar [31]	2003	Spain	25 AD	Cross-sectional	21.9 ± 13.3 mg/day	No correlation was found
Koetz [8]	2012	Germany	122 AD	Cross-sectional	21.9 ± 4.9 mg/day	No correlation was found
Chandy [34]	2016	India	41 AD	Cross-sectional	13.0 ± 3.0 mg/m^2	No correlation between daily glucocorticoid dose and low BMD.

Study, reference number	Year	Country	Population	Study design	HC dose	Impact of glucocorticoid dose on BMD
Schulz [5]	2016	Germany	90 AD	Prospective	30.8 ± 8.5 mg/day	A decrease in daily glucocorticoid dose from 30.8 mg to 21.4 mg induced a significant improvement in BMD at both lumbar spine and femoral neck sites.
Camozzi [32]	2018	Italy	87 AD	Cross-sectional	35 mg/day	
Our study	2021	Tunisia	50 AD	Cross-sectional	27.4 ± 6.7 mg/day CD:374.636 ± 283.821 mg 5924 ± 4648 mg/kg	Significant correlation between daily and cumulative dose and low BMD

Abbreviation: Hc, hydrocortisone; BMD, home mineral density; AD, Addison disease; CD: cumulative dose.

Table 6.
Synopsis of main clinical studies assessing the impact of glucocorticoid dose on BMD in patients with AD.

5. Conclusions

Glucocorticoid replacement therapy in AD may induce bone loss. Identification of predictive factors of low BMD in patients with AD is useful in the management of long-term glucocorticoid therapy's bone impact.

Thus, glucocorticoid therapy must be adjusted to the lowest-tolerable dose and regular measurement of bone mineral density may be useful to identify patients at risk for the development of osteoporosis.

Finally, further studies are needed to better analyze these factors and control BMD during the course of AD.

Acknowledgements

We appreciate the cooperation of all patients who participated in this study, especially during the COVID-19 pandemic.

Author contributions

Khouloud Boujelben: Conceptualization (equal); data curation (equal); formal analysis (equal); investigation (equal); methodology (equal); project administration (equal); validation (equal); writing – original draft (equal); writing – review and editing (equal). **Dhouha Ben Salah:** Data curation (equal); formal analysis (equal); methodology (equal); validation (equal); writing – original draft (equal).

Conflict of interest

No author has any conflict of interest.

Author details

Dhouha Ben Salah* and Khouloud Boujelben
Department of Endocrinology Diabetology, Hedi Chaker Hospital, Sfax University, Tunisia

*Address all correspondence to: bs.dhoha@gmail.com

References

[1] Øksnes M, Ross R, Løvås K. Optimal glucocorticoid replacement in adrenal insufficiency. Best Practice & Research. Clinical Endocrinology & Metabolism. 2015;**29**(1):3-15

[2] Isidori AM, Arnaldi G, Boscaro M, Falorni A, Giordano C, Giordano R, et al. Towards the tailoring of glucocorticoid replacement in adrenal insufficiency: The Italian society of endocrinology expert opinion. Journal of Endocrinological Investigation. 2020; **43**(5):683-696

[3] Hardy RS, Zhou H, Seibel MJ, Cooper MS. Glucocorticoids and bone: Consequences of endogenous and exogenous excess and replacement therapy. Endocrine Reviews [Internet]. 2018;**39**(5) Available from: https://pubmed.ncbi.nlm.nih.gov/29905835/

[4] Briot K, Roux C. Corticosteroid-induced osteoporosis. La Revue de Médecine Interne. 2013;**34**(5):315-323

[5] Schulz J, Frey KR, Cooper MS, Zopf K, Ventz M, et al. Reduction in daily hydrocortisone dose improves bone health in primary adrenal insufficiency. European Journal of Endocrinology. 2016;**174**(4):531-538

[6] Zelissen PM, Croughs RJ, van Rijk PP, Raymakers JA. Effect of glucocorticoid replacement therapy on bone mineral density in patients with Addison disease. Annals of Internal Medicine. 1994; **120**(3):207-210

[7] Braatvedt GD, Joyce M, Evans M, Clearwater J, Reid IR. Bone mineral density in patients with treated Addison's disease. Osteoporosis International: A Journal Established as Result of Cooperation Between the European Foundation for Osteoporosis and the National Osteoporosis Foundation of the USA. [Internet]. 1999; **10**(6). Available from: https://pubmed.ncbi.nlm.nih.gov/10663342/

[8] Koetz KR, Ventz M, Diederich S, Quinkler M. Bone mineral density is not significantly reduced in adult patients on low-dose glucocorticoid replacement therapy. The Journal of Clinical Endocrinology and Metabolism. 2012; **97**(1):85-92

[9] Proctor DN, Melton LJ, Khosla S, Crowson CS, O'Connor MK, Riggs BL. Relative influence of physical activity, muscle mass and strength on bone density. Osteoporosis International: A Journal Established as Result of Cooperation Between the European Foundation for Osteoporosis and the National Osteoporosis Foundation of the USA. 2000;**11**(11):944-952

[10] Lespessailles É. Ostéodensitométrie: Intérêts dans la prise en charge de la fragilité osseuse. Imagerie de la Femme. 2020;**30**(4):165-170

[11] Paz-Pacheco E, Fuleihan GE, LeBoff MS. Intact parathyroid hormone levels are not elevated in glucocorticoid-treated subjects. Journal of Bone and Mineral Research : The Official Journal of the American Society for Bone and Mineral Research. 1995;**10**(11):1713-1718

[12] Mazziotti G, Angeli A, Bilezikian JP, Canalis E, Giustina A. Glucocorticoid-induced osteoporosis: An update. Trends in Endocrinology & Metabolism. 2006; **17**(4):144-149

[13] Caplan A, Fett N, Rosenbach M, Werth VP, Micheletti RG. Prevention and management of glucocorticoid-induced side effects: A comprehensive

review: A review of glucocorticoid pharmacology and bone health. Journal of the American Academy of Dermatology. [Internet]. 2017;**76**(1) Available from: https://pubmed.ncbi.nlm.nih.gov/27986132/

[14] Oshagbemi OA, Burden AM, Shudofsky KN, Driessen JHM, Vestergaard P, Krings A, et al. Use of high-dose intermittent systemic glucocorticoids and the risk of fracture in patients with chronic obstructive pulmonary disease. Bone. 2018;**110**: 238-243

[15] Rs W. Clinical practice. Glucocorticoid-induced bone disease. The New England Journal of Medicine. 2011;**365**(1) Available from: https://pubmed.ncbi.nlm.nih.gov/21732837/

[16] Hardy RS, Zhou H, Seibel MJ, Cooper MS. Glucocorticoids and bone: Consequences of endogenous and exogenous excess and replacement therapy. Endocrine Reviews. 2018;**39**(5): 519-548

[17] Qian X. Glucocorticoids - New Recognition of Our Familiar Friend. [Internet]. 2012. Available from: https://www.intechopen.com/books/undefined/books/2538

[18] Suzuki Y, Ichikawa Y, Saito E, Homma M. Importance of increased urinary calcium excretion in the development of secondary hyperparathyroidism of patients under glucocorticoid therapy. Metabolism. 1983;**32**(2):151-156

[19] Streicher C, Heyny A, Andrukhova O, Haigl B, Slavic S, Schüler C, et al. Estrogen regulates bone turnover by targeting RANKL expression in bone lining cells. Scientific Reports. 2017;**7**(1):6460

[20] R G, Js W. The effects of glucocorticoid replacement therapy on growth, bone mineral density, and bone turnover markers in children with congenital adrenal hyperplasia. The Journal of Clinical Endocrinology and Metabolism. 1997;**82**(12) Available from: https://pubmed.ncbi.nlm.nih.gov/9398689/

[21] Bentivegna G, Osella G, Pia A, Terzolo M. Effects on bone health of glucocorticoid replacement therapy in primary and secondary adrenal insufficiency: A review. Current Opinion in Endocrine and Metabolic Research. 2018

[22] Suliman AM, Freaney R, Smith TP, McBrinn Y, Murray B, McKenna TJ. The impact of different glucocorticoid replacement schedules on bone turnover and insulin sensitivity in patients with adrenal insufficiency. Clinical Endocrinology. 2003;**59**(3):380-387

[23] Schafer AL, Shoback DM. Hypocalcemia: Diagnosis and treatment. In: Feingold KR, Anawalt B, Boyce A, Chrousos G, de Herder WW, Dhatariya K, et al., éditeurs. Endotext [Internet]. South Dartmouth (MA): MDText.com, Inc.; 2000. Available from: http://www.ncbi.nlm.nih.gov/books/NBK279022/

[24] Arlt W, Allolio B. Adrenal insufficiency. Lancet London England. 2003;**361**(9372):1881-1893

[25] Romão VC, Canhão H, Fonseca JE. Old drugs, old problems: Where do we stand in prediction of rheumatoid arthritis responsiveness to methotrexate and other synthetic DMARDs? BMC Medicine. 2013;**11**:17

[26] Kechichian E, Ezzedine K. Vitamin D and the skin: An update for dermatologists. American Journal of

Clinical Dermatology. 2018;**19**(2):
223-235

[27] Heureux F, Maiter D, Boutsen Y, Devogelaer JP, Jamart J, Donckier J. Evaluation of corticosteroid replacement therapy and its effect on bones in Addison's disease. Annales d'Endocrinologie. 2000;**61**(3):179-183

[28] Leelarathna L, Breen L, Powrie JK, Thomas SM, Guzder R, McGowan B, et al. Co-morbidities, management and clinical outcome of auto-immune Addison's disease. Endocrine. 2010; **38**(1):113-117

[29] Løvås K, Gjesdal CG, Christensen M, Wolff AB, Almås B, Svartberg J, et al. Glucocorticoid replacement therapy and pharmacogenetics in Addison's disease: Effects on bone. European Journal of Endocrinology. 2009;**160**(6): 993-1002

[30] Braatvedt GD, Joyce M, Evans M, Clearwater J, Reid IR. Bone mineral density in patients with treated Addison's disease. Osteoporosis international : A Journal Established as Result of Cooperation between the European Foundation for Osteoporosis and the National Osteoporosis Foundation of the USA. 1999;**10**(6): 435-440

[31] Jódar E, Valdepeñas MPR, Martinez G, Jara A, Hawkins F. Long-term follow-up of bone mineral density in Addison's disease. Clinical Endocrinology. 2003;**58**(5):617-620

[32] Camozzi V, Betterle C, Frigo AC, Zaccariotto V, Zaninotto M, De Caneva E, et al. Vertebral fractures assessed with dual-energy X-ray absorptiometry in patients with Addison's disease on glucocorticoid and mineralocorticoid replacement therapy. Endocrine. 2018;**59**(2):319-329

[33] Florkowski CM, Holmes SJ, Elliot JR, Donald RA, Espiner EA. Bone mineral density is reduced in female but not male subjects with Addison's disease. The New Zealand Medical Journal. 1994;**107**(972): 52-53

[34] Chandy DD, Bhatia E. Bone mineral density in patients with Addison disease on replacement therapy with prednisolone. Endocrine Practice : Official Journal of the American College of Endocrinology and the American Association of Clinical Endocrinologists. 2016;**22**(4):434-439

[35] Björnsdottir S, Sääf M, Bensing S, Kämpe O, Michaëlsson K, Ludvigsson JF. Risk of hip fracture in Addison's disease: A population-based cohort study. Journal of Internal Medicine. 2011; **270**(2):187-195

[36] Lee P, Greenfield JR. What is the optimal bone-preserving strategy for patients with Addison's disease? Clinical Endocrinology. 2015;**83**(2):157-161

[37] Delaisse JM, Andersen TL, Kristensen HB, Jensen PR, Andreasen CM, Søe K. Re-thinking the bone remodeling cycle mechanism and the origin of bone loss. Bone. 2020;**141**: 115628

[38] Li SS, He SH, Xie PY, Li W, Zhang XX, Li TF, et al. Recent progresses in the treatment of osteoporosis. Frontiers in Pharmacology. 2021;**12**: 717065

[39] Valero MA, Leon M, Ruiz Valdepeñas MP, Larrodera L, Lopez MB, Papapietro K, et al. Bone density and turnover in Addison's disease: Effect of glucocorticoid treatment. Bone and Mineral. 1994;**26**(1):9-17

[40] Nowotny H, Ahmed SF, Bensing S, Beun JG, Brösamle M, Chifu I, et al.

Therapy options for adrenal insufficiency and recommendations for the management of adrenal crisis. Endocrine. 2021;**71**(3):586-594

[41] Peacey SR, Guo CY, Robinson AM, Price A, Giles MA, Eastell R, et al. Glucocorticoid replacement therapy: Are patients over treated and does it matter? Clinical Endocrinology. 1997;**46**(3): 255-261